1981

University of St. Francis
G 362.10425 F443
Field, John W.
G

W9-ADS-688

3 0301 00068240 7

GROUP PRACTICE DEVELOPMENT

A Practical Handbook

John W. Field

LIBRARY
College of St. Francis
JOLIET, ILL.

Aspen Systems Corporation
Germantown, Maryland
1976

"This publication is designed to provide accurate
and authoritative information in regard to the
Subject Matter covered. It is sold with the
understanding that the publisher is not engaged in
rendering legal, accounting, or other professional
service. If legal advice or other expert assistance is
required, the services of a competent professional
person should be sought." From a Declaration of
Principles jointly adopted by a Committee of the
American Bar Association and a Committee
of Publishers and Associations.

Copyright © 1976 by Aspen Systems Corporation

All rights reserved. This book, or parts thereof, may not be
reproduced in any form or by any means, electronic or
mechanical, including photocopy, recording, or any
information storage and retrieval system now known or
to be invented, without written permission from the
publisher, except in the case of brief quotations embodied
in critical articles or reviews. For information, address
Aspen Systems Corporation, 20010 Century Boulevard,
Germantown, Maryland 20767.

Library of Congress Catalog Card Number: 76-56948
ISBN: 0-912862-26-2

Printed in the United States of America

1 2 3 4 5

G
362.10425
F443

5-12-81   Publisher $32.58

To Coco

95700

Table of Contents

List of Tables and Figures vii
Preface xi

Chapter 1 — The Emerging System of Health Care.......... 1
              Revolution in the Health Care Industry....... 3
              Growth in the Medical Industry 18
              Future Dynamics......................... 22
              Group Practice........................... 23
Chapter 2 — Blueprint For Change....................... 29
              The Power Centers 29
              Legislation at Work...................... 31
              Blueprint for the Future 33
              Blueprint in Action 44
              Success or Failure 47
Chapter 3 — Strategy for Participation 51
              Physician Strategy 53
              Hospital Strategy 59
              Insurance Company Strategy.............. 62
              Service Company Strategy................ 63
              Financial Company Strategy 64
              Consulting Firms........................ 64
              Other Groups........................... 64
              Payers of Health Care.................... 65
              Practitioners of Health Care.............. 65
Chapter 4 — The Pros and Cons of Group Practice.......... 71
              Patient Advantages and Disadvantages 73
              Practitioner Advantages and Disadvantages .. 74
Chapter 5 — Anatomy of Group Practice 79
              Market................................. 80

		Operating Establishment	86
		Supply Sources	100
Chapter 6	—	**Alternative Structuring**	103
		Service Line Alternatives	105
		Organization Alternatives	112
		Fiscal and Financial Systems Alternatives	123
Chapter 7	—	**Development Planning and Implementation**	135
		New Enterprise Projects	137
		Basic Kinds of Planning	142
		Basic Styles of Implementation	158
Chapter 8	—	**Aids and Sources**	163
		Resources and Suppliers	164
		New Opportunities	175
Chapter 9	—	**Conclusion**	183
		The Public Good	187
		Physicians' Welfare	191
		The Welfare of Others	194
		Removing the Roadblocks	196
Appendix A	—	**Planning Tables**	201
Appendix B	—	**Planning Case**	237
Index			299

List of Tables and Figures

Table	1:1	— Major Causes of Death in the U.S. — 1900 vs 1970	5
Table	1:2	— Medical Groups in the U.S. — 1959-1974	6
Figure	1:1	— Supply/Payroll Ratios — All Industry vs Medical Industry — 1976	9
Table	1:3	— Estimated Medical Revenue Transactions by Enterprise Class — 1976	10
Table	1:4	— Cost of Disease in the U.S. — 1976	15
Table	1:5	— Cause of Death in the U.S. — 1974	16
Table	1:6	— Profile of Illness in the U.S. — 1976	17
Table	1:7	— Activity Limited Persons in the U.S. — 1969-1970	17
Table	1:8	— Man-Days Lost Due to Disability in the U.S. — 1970	18
Table	1:9	— Annual Cost of Certain Disorders in the U.S. — 1976	19
Table	1:10	— Medical Industry Growth	20
Table	1:11	— Analysis of $ Growth of Medical Services — 1950 to 1975	20
Table	1:12	— Output per Physician	21
Table	1:13	— Hospital Personnel per 100 Census — Community Hospitals	21
Table	1:14	— Hospital Economic Factors	22
Figure	2:1	— An Integrated Configuration	43
Figure	2:2	— A Federated Configuration	44
Table	4:1	— Estate Building Capability — 1976 Dollars	76
Table	5:1	— Demand for Medical Care, 1976	85

Figure   5:1   — Hierarchical Organization Structure. .   88
Figure   5:2   — Division of a Complex.   90
Figure   5:3   — Hierarchical Physical Structure   92
Table   5:2   — Location of Various Resource
                     Capabilities.   101
Table   6:1   — Limited vs Extended Care.   107
Table   6:2   — Clinic Size Criterion for Inhouse
                     Medical Support Services   109
Table   6:3   — Desired Information Systems
                     Characteristics.   112
Table   6:4   — Executive Structure Integrated vs
                     Federated Establishments.   114
Table   6:5   — Organization Features by Legal
                     Types of Enterprise   119
Table   6:6   — Prepayment Plan Variations   124
Table   6:7   — Tax-Exempt Fringe Benefits
                     and Costs.   129
Table   6:8   — Other Tax-Exempt Benefits
                     and Costs.   130
Table   6:9   — Financial Structure Matrix   132
Figure   7:1   — Planning Hierarchy   143
Figure   7:2   — Map of Hamilton, N.Y.   146
Table   7:1   — Estimated Population (000s)
                     Hamilton, N.Y.   146
Table   7:2   — Providers in Hamilton and
                     Surrounding Areas.   147
Table   7:3   — Hospitals in Hamilton and
                     Surrounding Areas.   147
Table   7:4   — Disorder Spells in
                     Hamilton (1975).   148
Table   7:5   — Health Services Delivered in
                     Hamilton (1975).   149
Table   7:6   — Estimated Cost of Illness in
                     Hamilton (1975).   149
Table   7:7   — City of Hamilton Health
                     Care Goals (1985).   150
Table   7:8   — Major Goals of Hamilton
                     Medical Park.   151
Figure   7:3   — Proposed Organization for
                     Hamilton Medical Park.   151
Table   7:9   — Proposed Services for Hamilton
                     Medical Park.   152

Figure   7:4   — Proposed Flow of Services and
                    Funds at Hamilton Medical Park ...   153
Table   7:10   — Proposed Staff for Hamilton
                    Medical Park...................   154
Figure   7:5   — Proposed Building for Hamilton
                    Medical Park...................   155
Table   7:11   — Hamilton Medical Park Project
                    Program Completed to Date   156
Table   7:12   — Hamilton Medical Park Project Program
                    for Completion in the Future   157
Table   7:13   — Hamilton Medical Park Proposed
                    Flow of Funds (Thousands of
                    1975 $s Annually)   159
Table   7:14   — Hamilton Medical Park Capital Group
                    Proposed Input and Payout of
                    Funds   160
Table   8:1   — Nonprimary Care and Suppliers,
                    1976 Dollars   166
Table   8:2   — Operating Support Services and
                    Suppliers, 1976 Dollars..........   167
Table   8:3   — Captive Medical Care Units of a
                    Ten-Primary Care Practitioner
                    Practice......................   168
Table   8:4   — Captive Nonmedical Units and Sources
                    of a Ten-Primary Care
                    Practitioner Practice   169
Table   8:5   — Basic Operating Resources and
                    Sources of a Ten-Primary Care
                    Practitioner Clinic, 1976 Dollars ...   170
Table   8:6   — Basic Development Resources and
                    Sources — Ten-Primary Care
                    Practitioner Clinic, 1976 Dollars ...   171
Table   8:7   — Financial Resources and Sources —
                    Ten-Primary Care Practitioner
                    Clinic, 1976 Dollars..............   173
Table   9:1   — Prevalence of Illness, 1976..........   188
Table   9:2   — Estimated Cost of Medical
                    Services, 1976.................   189
Table   9:3   — Annual Cost of Disease Comparison ..   192
Table   9:4   — Potential Capital Requirements for
                    Group Practice 1976-1985.........   195

Preface

The new American frontier includes a rebuilding of major industries. Evidently, imperfections in some industries are too many for casual remedy. Individual industries have grown to become small economic systems in themselves. Many are in difficulty and their problems apparently call for industry-wide solutions.

The older economy with millions of semiautonomous enterprises was efficient, adjustable and self-correcting. It readily responded to the forces of supply and demand that controlled prices and weeded out incompetent providers. The influence of demand in the free market place gave people what they wanted and allowed industry to thrive as the system continuously purged itself of inefficient producers.

As enterprises grew, a new order of efficiency was attained. Large-scale organization, systemization, and mass production provided great increase in the output of goods for a growing population. But the prosperity was accompanied by difficult problems. The growth of individual enterprises concentrated power in the hands of fewer individuals. Power, in turn, corrupted, and subsequently required controls as competitive enterprises became quasi-monopolistic. Many enterprises became so large that they virtually precluded competition. As a result, government got involved in free enterprise, first as a regulator, and later as a planner and developer of industry.

Government grew and went into the system until today when it is almost impossible to tell where private industry ends and government begins. Federal, state and local agencies are immersed in practically every industry, including health care. Twenty percent of the national work force is employed by government; and about 40% of expenditure for end items are made by the government sector of the economy. It is informative to follow the growth of government influence by its role as taxer and consumer. Up until the Civil War, it took from 5% to 10% of the pot, by the end of World War I, around 17%, by 1950, 25%, and by 1976, around 40%.

With government's involvement with business and the growth of corporations, traditional modes of capitalism became strained. A century ago enterprises were largely financed by individuals who were identified as owners. Now it is difficult to find anyone who has a major stake in a large business. Private capital has given way to institutional capital. Large corporations, which employ more than 50% of the work force, are almost public institutions, a far cry from the individual enterprises of yesterday. Corporation executives are not the free-wheeling, profit-making characters pictured in Communist literature. They are quasi-public figures, more like government officials than the tycoons of old.

All kinds of social problems have arisen with the new amalgamation of government and industry. Pressure groups have found they can get what they want by challenging the establishment. With the breakdown of traditional capitalism, they feel justified in challenging private enterprise. They ask: "Why should the captains of industry set social objectives? Why should they make the national priorities?"

Almost overnight society has broken into groups practicing the act of dissent. The blacks protest the white power structure, the women strike out against the men, youth against their parents, the elderly against the young, the incarcerated against the free, labor against capital and consumer against producer. The thrust of each group has one common theme: "Let's get our share, including reparations for past injustices." Whether justified or not, the goals are centered on redistributing what we have as opposed to producing more, a primary cause of inflation in this decade.

The social unrest has apparently made inroads on our capacity to produce. Drug addiction, crime, rebellion, and anti-establishment attitudes have resulted in decreased productivity, contributing to inflation and stagnation. Attacks on industry for pollution, poor quality of merchandise, etc., which may be justified, contribute to the morass. The result has been a prolonged business recession with inflation--a situation relatively new to America.

And so it seems that rugged capitalism is apparently at the end of the road. What will come next: Communism, Socialism, Peoples' Republic? Probably none of these systems will be adopted. To do so would mean a regression. It is not likely that the outstanding economy will emulate second-rate competitors. American capitalism has been unique, leading a life of its own. As it evolves, it will continue to be unique and well ahead of socialistic competitors.

Indeed, a new system is already taking shape, a kind of community capitalism. It is retaining many virtues of traditional capitalism even as it embraces and incorporates governmental functions of a quasi-socialistic nature. Apparently it is going to be a system of reconstructed industries with federal, state, and local governments working closely with the private sector of the economy to formulate community-oriented complexes financed by private and government capital.

In such an economy, the capability to prosper will likely be retained. A proper blend of centralization and decentralization is likely to evolve, avoiding the destructive elements of a completely uncontrolled society and of a bureaucracy. Government operating through three levels will probably set the common social goals and provide some of the guidelines within which the private sector will work. In this way, it should allow freedom for individual action so that pluralistic systems can evolve and constructive competition with rewards for accomplishment can survive.

The reconstruction of various industries is underway. Those industries which pose a critical problem will be changed first. In fact, the priority list is already being formulated in the public forum. The medical industry is slated to be one of the first to undergo reconstruction. A virtual blueprint already exists in public documents, and work has been started. By 1985, the job could be completed. The medical industry, unlike many others, was never fully industrialized. In fact, it was suited for industrialization until recently. As a consequence, it remains highly individualistic with vestiges of the cottage industry age of capitalism.

In the early 1960s, the medical industry was deluged with demands it could not meet. The federal government launched Medicare and Medicaid almost simultaneously. In states like New York and California, the industry was faced overnight with a 20% jump in demand for services that had previously been expanding at about 3% per year. Medical costs shot up and continued to climb, at times doubling and tripling the general inflation rate.

Then the critics emerged. Articles and press releases by the thousands pointed out weaknesses in the industry. Much attention was given to the lack of preventive medical care.

Finally, the power centers went to work. Joining the opinion makers in condemning the system, they soon began to offer plans. Today, almost every public group has a blueprint: HEW, Republicans, Democrats, AMA, AHA, and about twelve influential members of Congress. While plans differ in detail, most are alike in major provisions. Such diverse groups as the Presidential staff, Congress, the American Hospital Association, and some physicians agree sufficiently to provide a fair consensus of what should be done. The provisions in pending legislation and in HEW regulations can be formulated into a flexible but definite blueprint for restructuring the industry.

The government has created a system at all three levels for planning and developing the new medical system. Prototype medical centers have already been started and a hundred or more are being planned. HEW expects that thousands of centers will exist by 1985. It is giving out grants ranging from $25,000 to $250,000 for planning and developing health care centers, and for startup operations, grants amounting to $2 to $4 million per center.

What will be your part in the emerging system of medical care? This handbook shows how you might participate: how to oppose as well as take part in the movement. It provides background, spells out the blueprint, and shows how it is being implemented. But most important, it gives you a strategy for participating.

If you are a physician or a dentist about to join a group, expand your practice or protect it, the books tells you what to do and how to do it. It also contains valuable information for medical students considering solo versus group practice, and for hospital administrators contemplating a comprehensive health care center. Others who will find useful suggestions are clinics, insurance companies, drug companies, clinical laboratories, service corporations, contractors, consultants, and venture capitalists.

Potential sponsors for medical centers will also be interested in the handbook. In addition to medical practitioners, unions and industrial companies, public officials and civic-minded citizens may also sponsor medical centers.

The American medical system is a huge enterprise generating $130 billion of services yearly, more than 8% of the gross national product. It employs over 5 million people and has $100 billion in tangible assets. The job of rebuilding the industry will take $50 billion or more in resources and the special efforts of several hundred thousand people over the next decade. It could be the outstanding achievement of the next ten years.

Chapter 1
The Emerging System of Health Care

For the past ten years, the medical economy has been going through a rapid evolution which is building to a crescendo. The rate of change seems destined to continue for another ten years, until the industry has undergone a fairly complete reconstruction. Profound economic, social and technological influences are bringing about these changes. They can be charted and their effects projected, give or take a few years.

The ostensible changes are manifestations of major underlying movements that are reshaping the medical industry at a near revolutionary pace. Through complex interactions, the underlying movements are causing a burgeoning of group practices. It appears that the evolving system of health care will take group practice as its building block, just as the former system was built on solo practice.

As the medical system evolves, there are far-reaching effects on those involved. Patients are subjected to new kinds of care as medical practice is steadily altered. Suppliers of resources are challenged to provide goods and services to support the changing industry. For some, the impact has been traumatic. Patients paying for care face skyrocketing costs. Medical institutions are caught in an economic squeeze between the rising cost of resources and public reluctance to pay more for care. Some medical practitioners are forced into new kinds of practice in order to survive.

The impact has not been completely negative. Suppliers of medical resources are seeing their market expand; and patients are getting more and better care. Some institutions are finding new roles that are both challenging and remunerative. But most significant is the effect on physicians, dentists, and other practitioners. Technological advances and new resources make possible improved medical care. In spite of bureaucratic influences, physicians have an opportunity to

1

create better practices. Through close collaboration, practitioners and suppliers of medical resources are likely to build a better medical system in the next decade. As they understand one another's problems better, they will be able to render mutual assistance. The upshot will be group practices that give better care at lower unit costs, while maintaining the dignity and integrity of professional practitioners.

How the medical economy finally shapes up depends upon decisions that will be made by those individuals involved. Patients are already faced with a choice of the kind of health care insurance they get in accordance with the HMO Act — whether to choose care in a closed-panel HMO, a foundation, or in conventional care establishments. What they choose will make a big difference in the mix of care centers that will evolve. Moreover, legislation in the mill will not only further increase the influence of patient decisions but will in part channel those decisions into the kind of medical system desired by the influential lawmakers.

The decisions of health providers will also influence the industry and how it develops. Some practitioners are fighting the bureaucracy; others are opting out altogether, preferring to go out of practice rather than conform with new regulations. Those in an adversary role are helping to ameliorate or improve public regulation; while others — more sympathetic to public controls — are helping the bureaucracy fashion regulations.

Most important in the transition process are several hundred thousand physicians who must decide how to practice in the future. They are faced with a changing medical economy in which most present practices will not be able to survive. At the same time, they have at their disposal the means for creating better practices. What they decide could make a significant difference in the final outcome. Their decisions will hinge on thousands of individual strategies. As each practitioner faces the mounting problems of today, he will develop a strategy to meet them. Some will sell their practices; others will join groups or even remain in solo practice. The overall change will depend upon the sum total of the individual strategies adopted, which will also make an important difference in how the overall medical economy emerges, and more important, in the success or failure of the individual practitioner.

Strategy is the key. This handbook details the strategy that depends on knowledge of what is happening and how to deal with it. It discusses the strategy of developing a group practice. It reveals the options, describes the opportunities, and tells how to participate in the creation, enlargement, and improvement of group practice.

REVOLUTION IN THE HEALTH CARE INDUSTRY

Revolution may be an apt term for what is happening in the health care industry. Here are some of the facts that should be known by anyone seriously engaged in the industry:

Since 1965—

- Health care expenditures nationally have gone up 325% from $40 billion to $130 billion.
- As a share of gross national product (GNP), health expenditures went from 6% to slightly over 8%.
- Almost 10% of disposable income is spent on health care annually, and the proportion spent has been going up relentlessly for a generation.
- The price of medical care has virtually doubled.
- Care per person has gone up almost 50%. Measured in 1976 dollars, it has gone from $400 to $600 per person.
- Group practices amounting to about 4,000 in number have more than doubled, and physicians in group practice have increased two and one-half times until now nearly a third of all independent practitioners are in group practice.
- Annual outpatient visits have increased from 125 million to 275 million.
- Clinical laboratory tests have tripled, from 1.5 billion annually to 4.5 billion--from $12 per person to $40.

The trend continues. Some projections published by reputable forecasters in the medical field maintain that by 1985:

- Health care expenditures will double, from $130 billion annually to $260 billion.
- As a share of the GNP, they will rise further and taper off at about 10%.
- Care per person will increase about 20% in the next five years and taper off thereafter.
- Group practice will increase to include a majority of independent physicians.
- Ambulatory care will continue to grow, displacing much inpatient care.
- Preventive care will grow from an estimated 20% of all care provided to approximately 40%.
- Clinical laboratory tests will increase from 4.5 billion annually to 10 billion.

Sources: U.S. Statistical Abstract
American Medical Association
American Hospital Association

Underlying these changes are three interrelated factors: (1) the industrialization of medicine; (2) the federalization of medicine; and (3) the comprehensive care movement. These powerful modifiers of the existing system should be understood by those contemplating new roles in it.

Industrialization of Medicine

In 1971, the Secretary of Health, Education, and Welfare, Elliot Richardson, issued a widely quoted White Paper that described the American medical system as a cottage industry. The secretary was promoting the Health Maintenance Organization (HMO) concept at the time and he linked the typical solo practitioner with eighteenth century artisans who worked alone in their homes and shops. He took pains to convince the reader that group practice is better than solo practice, and that a government-touted HMO is the best kind of practice.

The secretary evidently exaggerated to make his case. But, he had a point in calling the medical economy a cottage industry. It had some of the trappings of a cottage industry and still does. Modern industrialization came to medicine rather late, and not until recently has it made a sizeable impact.

Back in 1900, medicine was practiced in a kind of cottage industry. Most physicians worked out of their homes. While other workers had largely congregated in industrial centers many years before, the medical practitioner had remained among his patients. When people got sick, he went to their bedsides to treat them. People were born at home, died at home, and spent most of their sick time there. Seldom did they go to a hospital. Visits to doctors' offices were scarce compared to doctors' visits to patients.

In 1900, it was essential that doctors live near their patients since the major health problem was infection. When a person became ill, he went to bed and sent for his physician. A fever could mean pneumonia or influenza, diseases with high fatality rates. Because doctors visited patients, travel time had to be kept down.

During the past seventy-five years, medical practice has grown out of the cottage industry stage of 1900 to become a semi-industrialized system. It will continue to industrialize during the next decade. Starting at the turn of the century, inroads were made on infection. By 1930 life expectancy went up 20%. During the '30s and '40s the use of antibiotics, sterilization, pasteurization, and vaccination significantly affected the practice of medicine.

Today, infection is no longer the primary cause of death in the United States. With its progressive eradication, life expectancy has continued to go up. People are living much longer than they did in 1900 (till about 71 years of age on the average today as opposed to 49 years of age then). Infection no longer dictates how medicine will be practiced. In fact, the entire practice of medicine changed significantly as the primary cause of death shifted from infection to cardiovasclar disease and malignant neoplasm, a shift that is indicated in the following table:

TABLE 1-1
Major Causes of Death in the U.S.
1900 vs 1970

| | DEATHS PER 100,000 | |
	1900	1970
Upper respiratory infection	215	46
Diarrhea	143	1
Childhood diseases	63	21
Other infection	52	4
Total	473	72
Cardiovascular disease	256	500
Malignancies	64	162
Total	320	662

Source: Department of Commerce

By the end of World War II, a dramatic shift had taken place. Instead of the doctor visiting the patient as a rule, the patient went to the doctor. Physicians began to practice more effectively. They saved time by not traveling to see patients, by seeing them in their offices and learning to process several patients concurrently by diligent use of multiple examination rooms and staff assistants.

The new methods of practice provided more treatment. Patient visits per physician nearly doubled in the postwar period. Gradually, more paramedical and clerical assistants were employed, more outside supplies and services were used, and more equipment was acquired to examine and treat patients. These changes were part of the industrialization process.

As resources per physician grew, the need for additional space grew. Physicians pulled out of their homes and set up practice in professional office buildings. Soon they started sharing services on a significant scale. They shared space, receptionists, switchboard services, and other support services. Today many professional office buildings have stat labs, pharmacies, and radiologists — conveniently at hand for resident practitioners. Others provide a full range of services, including stenography, billing, and bookkeeping.

Ultimately, this congregation and progressive sharing led to group practice. Some physicians put it all together to form clinics. Starting as a trickle in 1950, the formation of clinics has grown progressively, as shown below. Many forecasters project more and larger group practices until 1985 when about 60% of independent practitioners, or twice today's number are projected to practice in groups.

TABLE 1-2
Medical Groups in the U.S. 1959-1974

Year	Medical Groups
1959	1,546
1965	4,289
1969	6,162
1976[1]	9,000

Note: [1]Estimated by the author
Source: Medical Groups in the U.S. 1969 by Todd & McNamara, published
       by the American Medical Association

Hospitals are also being industrialized. As the mix of diseases changed (heart disease and cancer displaced infection, and accident treatment increased), hospitals grew in importance. From simple charity homes for impoverished sick people, hospitals became complexes that serve as major medical centers. Many physicians have taken up practice in or around hospitals, and most physicians use hospitals as annexes to their office practices. Almost everyone is born in a hospital, many die there, and most serious spells of illness are treated in one.

In 1900, a hospital bed could be financed for less than $1,000. Today the investment cost is $150,000 per bed, and in some teaching hospitals, nearer to $200,000. The cost of running hospitals this year will be over $50 billion, in contrast with 1950, when it was $4 billion.

The modern hospital has come a long way in the process of industrialization. It is not only highly capitalized, but uses sophisticated equipment such as $400,000 clinical chemistry analyzers, $150,000 electronic microscopes, and $500,000 computers. It purchases large quantities of supplies and services from other industries. Many hospitals today are undergoing a crisis: they are too costly, and as new methods of practice evolve, the need for conventional hospital services is declining. It appears that in the next few years, many hospitals will take on new roles or go out of business.

The major limitation to the industrialization process both in hospitals and in office practice has been the need to keep physicians physically accessible to patients. Although the abatement of infection allows physicians to practice further away from patients, there are practical limits to the distances between them. Such limits tend to keep practices small, especially within rural areas. As physicians congregate into progressively larger groups, the number of entry places in the medical system shrinks proportionately; and the fewer the entry places, the further patients must travel to reach doctors. This principle, apparently overlooked by prominent social planners, puts a floor on the number of practices that are needed to assure adequate national health care coverage, and a practical ceiling on the average size of clinics. A recent study indicates that at least 10,000 entry points are needed, and it follows that with an expected 250,000 practicing office physicians, the average clinic should have no more than 25 physicians to accommodate the necessary number of clinics.

Another limitation to the industrialization process is physicians' reluctance to practice together. Most solo practitioners are rugged individualists. Their desire to remain independent has been a deterrent to the formation of group practice. It is also a deterrent to the practical size of a group, since a few doctors in a small group might get along well, but many doctors in a large group are likely to conflict.

Despite these limitations, the movement to group practice and further industrialization of medicine, which is both a cause and effect of group practice, continues. The trend shows no sign of abatement; in fact, there are factors thrusting the movement forward, such as patient preference, opportunity for improved care, and several economic influences.

One impelling factor involves the complexity of modern medicine. Since medicine is so complex a discipline, doctors have had to specialize. The combination of specialization and solo practice has raised different problems — not the least being where a patient goes for primary care or general advice on his health. Finding a primary care physician has become increasingly difficult, to the consternation of many patients. This has given rise to the solution of *one-stop care:* one place where a patient receives all the care needed.

Another curious feature of the system is that in solo practice the end product is often highly specialized, while those who provide the supporting services to the physician, because they are few in number, must be factotums performing a variety of chores. Since factotums are costly and their output, due to a lack of specialization, is small, the cost of care is higher than it would be in efficiently managed group practices. These disadvantages can be partially alleviated in a group practice where there is less shuffling of patients from one specialist to another, and the cost of support services can be reduced.

Another area of industrial thrust is medical supplies. The goods and services of other industries are playing an increasing part in the medical industry. In addition to equipment mentioned, the medical industry is using drugs, reagents, disposables, and services of other industries to improve medical care, increase output, and keep costs from increasing more rapidly. Today, 40% of the health care dollar goes to suppliers of goods and services.

A good indicator of the degree to which an industry is industrialized is the ratio of workforce earnings to supply expenditure. In industry as a whole, as shown below, the ratio is 35:65; in the medical industry, it is 60:40. The following figure shows that the medical industry is more than halfway along in catching up with other industry in the industrialization process.

The proportion of outside services and supplies that go into the medical care dollar is growing each year, and a recent study predicts that by 1985 the proportion will be 50% or more. Only the services of health care professionals are necessary to the industry; all the rest can be purchased today, which makes the potential use of supplies great. This has two implications: it represents an opportunity for medical suppliers, and it gives medical practitioners an opportunity to build systems largely on proven sources of outside supply in lieu of payroll services.

In the past, a major deterrent to industrialization was the fact that medicine is a service industry. Service industries, generally speaking, have been slow to industrialize. However, the situation is changing as some service industries — especially those that use the computer — find ways to industrialize. Health care is a knowledge producing industry, since 75% or more of medical effort is involved directly with some kind of information processing. Examination, diagnosis, prognosis, and to a

FIGURE 1-1: Supply/Payroll Ratios-All Industry vs. Medical
Industry-1976

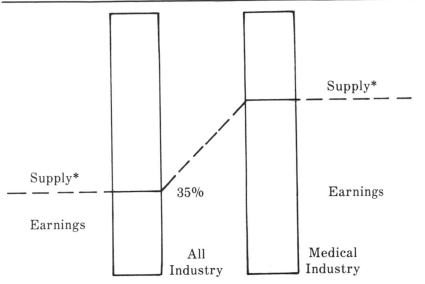

*Including all expenditures other than earnings, including investment costs.

large extent, treatment are knowledge and information processing functions; and the computer is becoming indispensable to all three. In the near future, excellence of medical care will probably depend almost as much on computer capacity, excellence of computer programs, and data banks, as it will upon the calibre of the professional staff in a clinic.

The computer not only aids in the creative aspects of care, but is also becoming indispensable in routine information processing. It is making inroads in booking, billing, and bookkeeping. As much as 30% of all employee time is being devoted to routine information processing. The table on the following page illustrates this point.

The health care industry is projected to provide some 7.0 billion service items in 1976. For each of these items there are at least three other information transactions that must be recorded, including the preparation of insurance and other claim documents required by public agencies and third parties. It is interesting to note that while some medical procedures cost thousands of dollars, the typical item of service costs only about $15. Since the paperwork cost of myriads of $15

TABLE 1-3
Estimated Medical Revenue Transactions by Enterprise Class–1976

Establishment Class	Revenue Transactions (Billions)
Hospitals	1.5
Nursing homes	0.1
Physician offices	1.4
Dental offices	0.5
Retail pharmacies	2.0
Other retail	0.5
Independent labs	0.5
Other	0.5
Total	7.0

Source: JFCo Estimate

items is huge, it appears that without the computer, paper shuffling could become the incubus of the medical industry.

Although industrialization has come to the medical industry late, it is making up for lost time. It will allow professionals in the industry to extend their medical capabilities, and in a partnership with medical suppliers build a stronger medical system.

Federalization of Medicine

All three levels of government have played a major role in health care. In recent years, governmental roles have grown. Now, largely under the aegis of the federal government, they have become almost dominant. More than 45% of medical revenues originate in tax dollars. Outside of industrialization, nothing has more influence on development of the medical industry than the part government plays, especially the federal government.

Government has played an important role in the medical industry since Revolutionary Days. It has protected the public from quacks by licensing, and from harmful drugs by the Pure Food and Drug Act. It has attempted to protect the consumer with price regulations. It has been researcher and sponsor of medical research, and one of the major providers of medical care through county, municipal, and federal hospitals, the Veterans Administration, and the military service. In addition to providing care directly, government has paid for care provided in the private medical industry— through Medicare, Medicaid, other welfare programs, and health care programs for government employees. It has helped finance a large part of the medical system that exists today. Government spends more than $55 billion annually for medical care. This amount not only increases each year, but the government's share of total medical expenditures also goes up.

The main thrust of federalization started in the '30s when health insurance took hold in a significant way. Though the system is a private one, the impact of health insurance on medicine and the overall economy has been so great it has been subject both to federal policy and state control under insurance laws. Approximately $40 billion annually is spent on health care through the private insurance system. Between federal expenditures and private insurance payments, the medical industry gets around 70% of its revenues from third parties.

Economists point out that private health insurance encourages overuse of medical services and is, therefore, a prime contributor to the continuing inflation of medical costs, another condition inviting federal controls. Over 80% of private insurance costs are borne by employers who have no control over medical use. They in turn pass these costs on to consumers just as taxes are tacked on to the cost of consumer goods. Concurrently, there is little incentive for the patient to cut down on care as his insurance policy covers most of it. Furthermore, he relies on his physician to decide whether care is necessary or not.

Physicians, in turn, have no incentive to economize on care. The decisions of a physician alone have no effect on what his patients pay out of pocket. Indeed, the contrary holds: there is a strong incentive to overuse medical services, especially where the physician is providing the services or has an interest in institutions providing them. The result is a national system in which the decision makers are not only not accountable for costs incurred but stand to personally benefit from them, a system in which expenses incurred are passed on to the general public in the form of a quasi-tax. It seems difficult to conceive of a more wasteful and inflationary system. Yet everyone went along with it for some time — until the cost of health care reached disturbing proportions. At that point, the federal government intervened.

Another precursor of federalization was the charitable role of hospitals. Originally, hospitals took care of the poor, the mentally ill, and patients with long-term illnesses such as tuberculosis. As medicine became industrialized and hospitals became the chief centers of care, state institutions continued to take care of the mental and tubercular patients, while short-term hospitals took on most of the rest. The short-term hospitals also continued to care for the poor suffering from acute illness, and a large part of their budgets went into such care. As they performed their charitable role, they relied on private and public grants for plant and equipment. However, the demand for hospital beds grew rapidly in the '30s and '40s. Not only was the medical industry turning to hospitals as it industrialized, but eradication of infection extended the age of the population, and as the proportion of older people grew, bed days per person correspondingly increased. This continued until after World War II, when the demand for hospital beds could not be met under the older system of charity financing. The federal government stepped in, giving grants and other assistance with the passage of the Hill-Burton Act in 1946.

Hill-Burton helped finance about half of the existing short-term hospital beds. But more important, it led to areawide planning legislation that may ultimately have more influence on medicine than Hill-Burton itself. In 1962, areawide planning legislation was passed at the federal level. Since then, there has been an attempt to control construction of medical facilities via a hierarchy of planning agencies at all three levels of government.

Areawide planning legislation has been augmented and strengthened several times, giving the original legislation more jurisdiction and teeth to enforce the will of planning agencies. The Health Planning Act of 1975 was the latest move to strengthen areawide planning; and if it goes as planned, the medical industry will be treated like a utility — with everyone seeking approval of a local commission in order to set up or change practice. There is still, however, considerable question whether the new legislation has the clout to do what its advocates want. Apparently, a bill with the necessary teeth could be declared unconstitutional.

Areawide planning is rooted in the concept that medicine is a public utility and, therefore, needs regulation of a public utility nature. There are many arguments in the public forum to support this case. It is contended, for example, that duplication of expensive facilities raises the cost of care unnecessarily and leads to ruinous competition. But there are also strong arguments against the case — notably, that regulation creates more costs than it saves, that medicine is more like conventional industry than utilities, and that restricting competition with regulation does more harm than good. As the issue is joined, government officials are attempting to erect stronger control agencies, while influential private agencies are opposing them. It should be a long struggle ultimately resolved by the courts.[1]

From 1950 to 1965, medical care increased nearly 100%, almost 50% per person, as more care was extended to the indigent and the aged, and because of the charity burden hospitals undertook a Robin Hood role by overcharging those able to pay in order to subsidize the poor. In addition, the United Fund and other eleemosynary systems were cranked up to supply deficit-financing for hospitals until the entire medical economy came under great strain. Then Medicare and Medicaid programs got underway to bail out the hospitals. They have become essential sources of revenues ever since.

As Medicare and Medicaid abuses were visibly increasing, the federal government stepped in and passed PSRO legislation in 1973. Thus another big step was taken in the federalization of medicine. PSRO not only set standards for delivery and payment of care under federal programs, but by suasion extended such controls to all kinds of care. Along with passage of PSRO legislation, the federal government passed the HMO Act — perhaps the most significant legislation in the federalization process. This act prescribes a favored form of medical care organization — the health maintenance organization (HMO). It gives HMOs favored treatment not only in the ways of grants and financing but in a provision that could ultimately drive out other kinds of care centers. That provision mandates that employers of 25 people or more, who pay for health care as a part of employee reimbursement, give employees the option of joining a government approved HMO. This unusual privilege is about to be tested in the courts and may ultimately be found unconstitutional. More likely, before this happens, the privileges extended to HMOs will be given to other kinds of practice.

The definition of an HMO under the law is both complex and incomplete. It is incomplete in the sense that implementation of the law calls for progressive refinement of the definition, which is now happening. In proximate terms, an HMO is an HEW-approved health care organization that gives a fairly comprehensive range of care to enrollees for prepaid annual fees.

HMOs have been around for about half a century under different names. The Kaiser Health Organization is the outstanding one today and, interestingly enough, the largest private medical care organization in the world. The proponents of HMOs are convinced that they can give superior medical care, and that they can improve the health of persons enrolled while also reducing health care costs through preventive care. They cite convincing statistics, but have not proved their case, at least not to a large number of antagonists.

Many medical economists and government officials believe that the prepaid feature of HMOs, sometimes called the capitation method, is the only way to remedy inflation built into the existing medical care insurance system. In the prepayment method, the physicians of a clinic are paid a flat amount per head each year for all the enrollees in the clinic. For the flat sums paid, the clinic must provide all the care that is needed for all its enrollees without further charge or assessment except for minor surcharges which may be allowed. And this includes payment for essential services of specialists and institutions outside of the health care organization.

Under such circumstances, there is both an incentive to keep patients well and to use both prudence and restraint in the use of services. There is no incentive for overuse as there is under the current system, since overuse comes out of the expenses of the clinics involved and eventually out of the pockets of physicians making the treatment decisions. In this way, the capitation method of paying for medical services does make the physician more accountable for his decisions, introducing responsibility into the decision-making process. For these reasons, capitation is frequently cited as the foremost feature of HMOs. The goal of extending capitation methods of payment along with HMOs has become part of the federalization process.

All of the pieces except one have been put in place for a federalized system of medicine. The one remaining is a national health insurance program (NHI), which legislators have been working on for more than five years. There are scores of bills in Congress on this subject. Some are in their third and fourth major revisions. Several would nationalize medicine with the federal government paying the bill for all medical care. Others fall considerably short of nationalization; but all are significant bills that call for major changes in the existing health system.

The chances of passage of a sweeping act that virtually nationalizes the medical system seem to be waning. While nothing is certain in politics, long-range trend away from government regulation is appearing, which should augur well for a moderate form of national health insurance. Further delay of several years or more before passage of NHI is also possible. In the meantime, the medical industry will go a long way in reconstructing itself to meet national health care goals.

Comprehensive Care Movement

As industrialization and federalization of health care go on, medical care is becoming more comprehensive, a trend with far-reaching influence on the medical economy. Care by crisis is being augmented with arrestive care of a high order, rehabilitative care, and preventive care. Furthermore, the definition of disease is expanding to include disorders such as alcoholism, drug addiction, obesity, and depression. As the disease horizon expands, new procedures are devised to diagnose and treat the newly classified disorders. In the comprehensive care movement, the growth of preventive care is crucial. Improved health monitoring procedures and educational aids are making it possible to prevent and delay many diseases.

The economic impact of the comprehensive care movement is enormous — not just on the medical economy alone but on the overall economy and the social well-being of the nation. Curious sets of cause and effect factors exist in which the comprehensive care movement interacts with the other major movements, the industrialization and federalization of medicine. It is both a cause and result of industrialization, and a cause and result of federalization.

Another curiosity, and an anomaly, is the relationship between comprehensive care and eradication of infection. As acute illness is eradicated, per capita care requirements go up rather than down, as might be expected. This comes about in part because of an aging population due to the eradication of acute illness itself. As acute cases get eradicated they are replaced by chronic ones that require more care per illness. Care requirements increase because of the broader definition of disease, the broader horizons of effective treatment, and new opportunities to improve life quality through health care. In a benign way, the medical industry is expanding its own market.

The cost of health in the United States, or more precisely the lack of health, is roughly $360 billion annually — divided among the costs of care, premature death, and disability as shown below.

TABLE 1-4
Cost of Disease in the U.S.A.—1976

ITEM	ANNUAL COST ($Bil)
Premature death	85
Disability and Incapacity	145
Medical care	130
Total	360

Source: JFCo Staff Study

A recently published study puts the economic cost of premature death at $85 billion annually. It excludes, of course, the grief associated with death. The study was predicated on a full life-span of 80 years. It tallied the productive losses of net national product in the future due to premature death, and the sums derived were converted to present dollar values in an appropriate cash-flow discounting procedure.

Diseases in relatively few categories account for almost all death at this time, as shown below. All the diseases listed have preventive regimens. Many medical authorities believe that the incidence of the acute diseases shown can be further reduced, and that the incidence of the chronic ones can be postponed. If so, this would reduce premature death.

TABLE 1-5
Cause of Death in the U.S.A.—1974
(Total Deaths - 1,950,000)

CAUSE OF DEATH	PERCENT OF TOTAL
Heart disease	38
Cancer	17
Stroke	11
Accidents & violence	8
Respiratory infection	4
Other arterial	3
Diabetes	2
Cirrhosis of the liver	2
Early diseases of infants	2
Other infection	2
Emphysema	1
All other	10
Total	100

Source: Statistical Abstract of the U.S.

Americans are afflicted with more than 500 million spells of illness each year, about 2-1/2 spells per person. The spells are largely due to short-term illness that responds quickly to treatments administered in one or two office visits. Initial spells of long-term or chronic illness are much less frequent. However, most of these cases carry over from year to year, often snowball, and frequently require repetitive office visits over many years. A profile of illness is shown in Table 1-6.

TABLE 1-6
Profile of Illness in the U.S.A.—1976

TYPE OF DISORDER	INCIDENCE — MILLIONS ANNUALLY		
	NEW	CONTINUING	TOTAL
Episodic			
Respiratory illness	240	-	240
Accident	70	-	70
Other infection	50	-	50
Digestive illness	25	-	25
Pregnancy	2	-	2
Continuing*			
Heart disease	2	20	22
Muscle, joints & bone DO	2	26	28
Mental & addictions	2	36	38
Hypertension	1	18	19
Cancer	0.7	1	1.7
Diabetes	0.3	8	8.3
Total	395	109	504

*A continuing illness is counted as one spell per year
Source: JFCo Study

In addition to spells of illness, more than 20 million people are more or less permanently disabled, as shown in Table 1-7.

TABLE 1-7
Activity Limited Persons in the U.S.A.–1969-70

DISABILITY	ACTIVITY LIMITED PEOPLE	
	MILLION	% OF POPULATION
Heart conditions	15.5	7.8%
Arthritis & rheumatism	14.1	7.0
Visual impairment	4.8	2.4
Hypertension (alone)	4.6	2.3
Mental & nervous conditions	4.5	2.3
Total limitations	43.5*	-
Total persons	23.2	11.7

*Includes multiple limitations per person
Source: U.S. Statistical Abstract

According to the U.S. Statistical Abstract, time lost in illness amounts to three billion man-days annually, as shown in the next table. The productive value of man-days lost and the loss of efficiency due to handicap amount to around $145 billion annually — about 10% of the GNP.

TABLE 1-8
Man Days Lost Due to Disability in the U.S.A.—1970

CONDITION	TIME IN BILLIONS OF MAN-DAYS
Bed restriction	1.2
Recuperation after hospital	0.2
Other restriction	1.6
Total	3.0

Source: U.S. Statistical Abstract

The remaining $130 billion is for care itself, which brings the total up to $360 billion annually — almost 25% of the GNP. The cost of disease is apparently one of the major factors in the overall economy; the ravages of disease are among the chief detractors of life quality in our society.

Comprehensive care promises not only to reduce the ravages of disease — possibly to eliminate most of it in time — but to significantly improve the quality of life by occupational enhancement, leisure time enhancement and life extension.

The following table shows the annual cost of twelve types of physical disorders that in aggregate cost around 20% of the GNP annually and detract from the quality of life (in effort, grief, and incapacitation) by much more than that amount.

Since comprehensive care is making inroads in these diseases, the costs will continue to grow.

GROWTH IN THE MEDICAL INDUSTRY

The trio of underlying movements — industrialization, federalization, and the comprehensive care movement — account for the near revolutionary changes in the medical industry. In the period 1950-1975 medical expenditure adjusted for price change went up about three

TABLE 1-9
Annual Cost of Certain Disorders in the U.S.A.—1976

DISEASES	SUFFERERS[1] (MILLION)	ANNUAL COST ($ BILLION)
Acute illness	10	60
Heart disorder	20	50
Accidents & violence	2	30
Alcoholism	10	20
Psychiatric disorder	4	20
Cancer	1	20
Tension, anxiety, depression	22	15
Muscle, joint, bone DO	27	15
Other addiction	1	12
Hypertension (severe)	18	10
Diabetes	8	8
Obesity	50	7
Total	90[2]	282

[1] At a given time.
[2] Does not add because of multiple disorders per person.
Source: JFCo Analysis of various newspaper clippings

times, and still continues to rise dramatically. The 3.0 times increase was accomplished with only a 1.5 times increase in the physician workforce, and was administered to a population that increased only 1.4 times. Indeed, the care expenditure per person in the population, adjusted for inflation, grew 2.25 times. Table 1-10 is a tabular profile of these changes.

In actual dollars, growth was even more spectacular because of price increases of more than 3.0 times. For example, in 1950 expenditures were only $12 billion compared with $118 billion in 1975—a growth of nearly ten times. An analysis of total growth, including price factors involved, is shown in Table 1-11.

Physicians just about doubled their efficiency in the 1950-1975 period. They did it by reducing house calls, creating more effective office procedures, employing industrial aids, etc.

TABLE 1-10
Medical Industry Growth

Fiscal Year	Expenditure 1975 ($ billion)	Physicians (thousand)	Population (million)	Index of Expenditure Per Person
1950	37	233	152	100
1955	43	255	166	
1960	52	274	181	
1965	70	305	194	
1970	91	348	205	
1975	118	390	215	225

Source: U.S. Statistical Abstract (extended)

TABLE 1-11
Analysis of $ Growth of Medical Services
1950 to 1975

Due to increased population	1.42
	x
More care per person	2.25
	x
Price increase	3.08
Equals the overall change	9.83

Source: U.S. Dept. of Commerce (extended)

Hospitals also expanded their service output, though not uniformly. Long-term hospitals have been gradually fading out as better treatment for tuberculosis and serious mental disorders is developed, while short-term hospitals, especially community hospitals, are increasing.

Between 1950 and 1975 demand for hospital services went up more than 2.0 times, while beds increased only 5%. To meet the increased demand with the limited number of beds, services per bed went up 1.9 times. Progressively more personnel per patient day was required by

TABLE 1-12
Output per Physician

YEAR	INDEX
1950	100
1960	123
1970	170
1975	195

Source: JFCo Analysis

community hospitals to provide expanding services, as indicated below:

TABLE 1-13
Hospital Personnel per 100 Census—Community Hospitals

YEAR	INDEX
1950	84
1960	114
1970	196
1975	240E*

Source: Hospital Statistics

In the 1950-1975 period, services performed by all hospitals expanded from $4 billion annually to $48 billion. The mean charge per patient day went from $8 to $90.

---

*For purposes of this book, the letter "E" represents estimate.

Inflation accounted for most of the change. When the figures are corrected for it, the resultant increase in output was 2.0 times. Applied to a population that grew 1.4 times, the increase per person in the population was 1.42 times. And due to a reduction in length of stay to meet burgeoning hospital demand, along with an increased work load per stay, the output per patient day went up 1.9 times. A profile of these changes is shown in the following table.

TABLE 1-14
Hospital Economic Factors

Fiscal Year	Hospital Services ($billion)	Charge Per Patient Day	Cost Index	Index of Output		
				Total	Per Person	Per Patient Day
1950	4	$8	100	100	100	100
1960	9	16				
1970	28	54				
1975	48	90	600	200	142	190

Source: JFCo Analysis of Dept. of Commerce Data

FUTURE DYNAMICS

The next decade will see the culmination of industrialization, federalization and the comprehensive care movement. The phenomenal growth rate of medical care should continue as the potential to improve the quality of life is exploited. The result would be more care per person for the moderately growing population--considerably more care in the aggregate. There will be more care per person, a moderately larger population, less acute disease, more elderly people, more chronic illness, more preventive care, less inpatient care and more ambulatory care.

The medical system will be strained to meet the growing and changing needs of the public. Hospitals are already feeling strain as ambulatory care displaces inpatient care. There is, and will continue to be, a tendency for medical costs to rise as more care per person, numbers of persons needing care, and unit costs of care go up.

At the same time, there is a limit to what people will pay for health care. With care costs running at 10% of disposable income, people are uneasy and somewhat resentful, according to public opinion samplings. Politicans who want to nationalize the system have stated that if medical costs get much higher, the public will clamor for nationalization. Meanwhile, demand for care continues to rise, and costs continue to go up as prices spiral.

The system is caught in a serious squeeze between demand and supply. It simply cannot supply all the care that is needed. Spiraling prices are a symptom of this situation. The big question is how the crisis will be resolved. Will nationalization of the industry take place? A further spate of government controls, including fee regulation? Or something less drastic? Whatever course is taken, a satisfactory solution will include some way to improve the productivity of the industry. In no other way can the needs of the public be met.

Fortunately, there appears to be a solution in group practice. The evidence is mounting that medical practitioners can work more effectively together than apart. By joining together they can afford facilities beyond the reach of solo practitioners. They can set up processing systems in which their employees can specialize efficiently. Group practice can exploit many industrial resources beyond the immediate reach of solo practitioners. It is also more conducive to the practice of comprehensive care.

For these reasons, the future dynamics of medicine will be tied up with group care. Reconstruction of the industry will involve creation of comprehensive care centers to handle most of the nation's health needs. If the private medical industry does not create them, the federal government will. It is almost certain, however, that both will play an important part, with the government creating further incentives to the private sector.

GROUP PRACTICE

A group practice is an association of three or more medical practitioners, made up of any combination of licensed physicians, engaged jointly in providing medical services. A solo practitioner is one who practices alone. The definition also excludes associations of two — usually two-man partnerships that function more like solo practices than groups.

In addition to the *three or more* qualification, the term *association* is important. There are many kinds of medical associations. Some are group practices, some are not. There are the legal or formal associations that qualify, such as corporations, cooperatives, and other chartered institutions; and there are partnerships of three or more practitioners that fit the broader definition of association. Finally, there are "loose" associations of practitioners sharing practice or resources with one another under a single name or "shingle." Not included in the definition, however, are otherwise independent practitioners who may share something, such as a nurse, office space, or other resource.

There are many kinds of group practice. For the moment we will confine ourselves to one classifying axis—the variety of care performed by groups. Using this classification, all groups can be sorted into one of two types—*single specialty* and *multispeciality*. Ten gynecologists or six pediatricians practicing together are examples of a single specialty group. An assortment of specialists, such as an internist, a general surgeon, a urologist, a psychiatrist, a dentist, and a general practitioner (also considered a specialist) constitute a multispecialty group.

Until recently, most of the growth in group practice has been in single specialty groups. After World War II, such groups were established for the treatment of specific disorders, such as cancer, psychiatric problems, and bone and pediatric diseases. The chief reason for this growth was the desire to acquire professional excellence in an association of peers.

Recently, the focus of growth has shifted to comprehensive health care organizations. These are multispecialty groups that give a full range of care to patients, as opposed to other multispecialty groups that give only limited care. The comprehensive groups try to be one-stop centers for all medical problems. They try to keep patients well in addition to treating illness. (See Chapter 2 for a discussion of CHOs.)

Today, nearly 30% of independent office physicians are in group practice. This increase from only a handful 20 years ago shows the rapid growth of group practice.

Underlying the growth are two sets of causes. First, more physicians prefer to practice in a group. Second, organizations outside the industry, particularly the federal government, are sponsoring and encouraging the formation of health care centers. In spite of the recent HMO fanfare, most of the group practice stimulus has come from within the private medical sector. The advantages of group practice apparently grow as the medical industry changes under the impetus of industrialization, federalization, and the comprehensive care movement.

Several hundred group practices, including some of the largest, got underway because communities, unions, companies, and governments were dissatisfied with the care available. The Kaiser Health Plan was started to bring health care to underserved areas prior to World War

II. Health Insurance Plan of New York, or HIP, was started in the late '30s to give medical services to employees of New York City and to provide a place of practice for immigrant physicians who were plentiful at that time. Group Health Association of Washington, D.C. was started in the '30s to care for federal employees. Neighborhood Health Associations and new HMOs have been sponsored and funded by the federal government recently to hold down the federal cost of care and to encourage a government-preferred kind of care organization.

While there are still few federally sponsored care centers, the federal program itself is a spur to the private sector. HMOs and other favored care centers are a threat to private practice. They can and do take patients away from private practitioners; and their competition has prompted some practitioners to go into group practice earlier than they might have. In addition, government regulations are becoming so complex, practitioners are seeking refuge in groups that can cope with them.

The shiftover from solo to group practice appears to be reaching lively proportions. A study published several years ago on group practice predicted this and concluded that most medical and dental practitioners will be in groups practicing comprehensive care by 1984. According to the study, there should be ten thousand comprehensive care centers by 1984, some independent, and some associated with hospitals.

Not all physicians welcome the trend. The growth of group practice is a threat to those who wish to remain in solo practice. Group practice itself, especially as it is portrayed by government sponsors, is anathema to many physicians. Some erroneously believe that they will find only salaried jobs in group practice, that they will be told how to practice by a superior, and that they will be tied up in red tape by an administrator. Their fears are partly justified in that many group practices are more administratively than professionally oriented; they stress hierarchy and centralization in organization rather than flexibility and decentralization, and emphasize interdependence rather than independence. These features, of course, are not essential in group practice; yet they prevail to the extent that they inhibit its growth.

Physicians and dentists don't have to become employees, working for crass businessmen, or worse yet, bureaucratic administrators. They need not advertise and ring doorbells to get patients as some bureaucratic plans prescribe. If they regulate themselves within reason, they need not be regulated by others—including fee regulations, as long as other prices of the free market are not regulated. They need not work for capitation—getting paid a flat annual fee to

95700   **LIBRARY**
College of St. Francis
JOLIET. ILL.

take care of a patient — but may stay with the fee-for-service method of payment. In short, they have many options today and in spite of threats heard in the public forum, it is likely that most of the options will remain.

Further, in an effort to get physicians into group practice, the government recently created some additional options in the form of tax incentives, financial aids, and other assistance. So, while preserving old options, physicians can capture new ones for developing better practice in the emerging system of health care.

There is, in fact, nothing to keep physicians and others from creating practices that combine most of the desirable features of solo practice with the advantages of group practice. Nothing, that is, except the knowhow and the desire. As practitioners become enlightened about group practice, discovering its varied possibilities and potential advantages, they become more prone to joining or creating groups. However, those who are proselytized or convince themselves to get into group practice don't always find it easy to do so. It takes careful search and investigation to find a compatible group; and more often than not, such a group does not exist for those seeking one. For those who can't find a satisfactory group, the alternative is to start one. But that is not an easy task, particularly for the practitioner who hasn't the knowledge of how to go about it.

Furthermore, the creation of a group practice takes a number of practitioners. Often it takes community cooperation and the resources of many suppliers. Besides doctors and dentists and other health care practitioners, the following kinds of people and agencies can be involved in creating a group practice:

- Prominent citizens and public officials for sponsorship
- Consultants to develop a business plan
- Lawyers for permits, contracts, etc.
- Accountants for records and tax counsel
- Insurance carriers for medical plans and risk coverage
- Architects for business plans
- Builders for facilities
- Venturers for risk capital
- Bankers for loans
- Equipment suppliers for hardware systems
- Investment counsel for estate building plans
- Hospitals and others for auxiliary health care support
- Other suppliers for goods and services
- Government people for cooperation and advice

The development of group practice is obviously multidisciplinary. It has many roles which are closely interrelated. As the medical industry is rebuilt on group practice, the individuals involved will interact closely with one another. Indeed, the speed and effectiveness of reconstruction will depend on how well the parties interact. The quicker practitioners get to know and work with other potential participants, the faster the job will be done. A key to success in the group practice movement, therefore, is how well the different participants understand one another's roles. To emphasize this, two prescriptions are suggested: (1) practitioners should understand the role of resource suppliers; and (2) suppliers should understand the role of practitioners.

The need for understanding reciprocal roles is a major controlling factor in the development of group practice. It will determine the speed at which the medical system responds to the public demand for more care at a reasonable cost. It also suggested the style of this handbook, in which the reciprocal roles are set forth for the briefing of all major participants in the group practice movement.

NOTE

1. The Supreme Court of South Carolina has already ruled against the public utility concept by declaring unconstitutional the stipulation of most planning agencies that a certificate-of-need be acquired from a state planning authority for medical facilities construction.

Chapter 2
Blueprint for Change

PUBLIC OPINION

Public opinion polls conducted over the last five years show that a majority of Americans want some kind of national health insurance system. Many express the desire for more preventive medicine, continuity of doctor-patient relationships, and a single place where they can go for care.

Public opinion has been molded by the media, which has been describing how bad American medicine is. Charges are repeatedly made that America ranks poorly among nations in life expectancy, infant mortality, and in other areas. Dissatisfaction over the rising costs and the unavailability of doctors is mounting as are complaints that doctors are too busy to practice preventive medicine.

But doctors have not had equal time to answer these charges with the counter-argument that: (1) social factors rather than inadequate care have more effect on health than the care system itself; (2) the stress and strain of our lifestyle is a major factor in American health status; and (3) the economics of preventive medicine are questionable. As a result, the argument has apparently been fought and won by the opinion makers.

THE POWER CENTERS

It takes more than public opinion to revolutionize an industry, particularly one large enough to generate $130 billion of services annually. Power centers are required, such as the administration, both the Democratic and Republican parties, the AHA, the AMA, and others. Such centers have been at work.

In July 1970, former HEW Secretary Elliot Richardson stated that "By the end of the decade the goal will be to have sufficient HMOs to enroll 90% of the population."

An article entitled "Meet the HMO" published in 1971 in *Changing Times* similarly stated that:

> ...a remarkably diverse group, including President Nixon, Congressional strategists, some private physicians and medical associations now consider HMOs as likely structures for bringing better health care to more people for less money.

Since these statements, more than a dozen bills for changing the medical delivery system have been before Congress. They represent diverse objectives and contributed to conflicts that could take many years to resolve. Yet the bills have much in common. Most call for national health insurance to cover everyone, not just for sick-care but for well-care, too.

The bills sponsored by organized labor and Senator Kennedy would provide the greatest scope of coverage, paid for by the federal government out of substantially increased taxes, in a system of health maintenance centers where physicians would essentially be quasi-government employees—much like they are in England today. Other bills with less coverage would rely on industry to pay care costs through the existing private insurance industry. For example, bills associated with Senators Long and Ribicoff and many associated with the Ford Administration limit coverage mainly to catastrophic care paid by private industry.

The AHA has a published plan for remodeling the medical system around what it calls health care corporations. According to an AHA pamphlet:

> The Health Care Corporation would synthesize management, physicians, personnel, and facilities into a corporate structure with the capacity and responsibility to deliver comprehensive health care to the community, either directly through its own facilities and services or by contract with other health care providers.

Finally, the American Medical Association has a plan called Medicredit which would provide universal health insurance through a system of income tax credits. This plan is before Congress in several bills. In addition, the AMA concedes that some good may come out of HMOs. In a paper dated May 1971, the Division of Medical Practice stated:

> To the HMO itself, the Association has no clear-cut policy objection. The AMA supports a pluralistic delivery system and

the right of both patient and physician to choose the system in which they both encounter each other, as long as that system exploits neither patient nor physician.

LEGISLATION AT WORK

The power centers have been doing more than talking — they have a blueprint, and a significant body of legislation already passed, and being implemented. Some of the significant legislation at work includes:

Hill-Burton Program. Hill-Burton grants which started in 1946 have financed much of the hospital construction of the past 30 years. Recent Hill-Burton amendments provide grants for outpatient facilities and diagnostic centers.

Comprehensive Health Planning and Public Health Services Act of 1966 (Public Law 89-749). This law created the Partnership for Health Program, a governmental system of health planning, which includes:

1. A national advisory council on comprehensive health planning programs.
2. State planning agencies (A-agencies).
3. Regional planning agencies (B-agencies). The agencies not only plan but control health facilities construction by certificate-of-need programs.

Professional Standards Review Organization Amendments of 1972 (Public Law 92-603). This law prescribes a nationwide professional standards review organization, PSRO, now in the process of being developed. The system, when it is fully operating, will consist of several hundred regional nonprofit organizations that will fit into a control hierarchy headed by HEW. It will:

1. Provide quality and cost standards for practitioners and centers handling Medicare and Medicaid patients.
2. Control entrance of Medicare/Medicaid patients into hospitals for surgery.
3. Audit Medicare and Medicaid bills.
4. Audit Medicare and Medicaid practice.
5. Take disciplinary action when justified.

The Health Maintenance Organization Act of 1973 (Public Law 93-222). This law defines in gross terms a health maintenance organization and sets up an administrative procedure for refining the definition and creating implemental regulations. The major feature of the act, dubbed by some a sleeper, is the following provision:

> *Sec 1310(a)* Each employer which is required during any calendar quarter to pay its employees the minimum wage. . ., and which during such calendar quarter employed an average number of employees of not less than twenty-five, shall . . . include in any health benefits plan offered to its employees . . . the option of membership in qualified health maintenance organizations. . .

The law provides federal grants and loan guarantees for several hundred new HMOs. But most important, through the sleeper provision, it establishes HMOs as a favored kind of health care establishment. Two kinds of HMOs are specified in the act. One is a so-called closed panel establishment where doctors work together as teams. The other is an open panel establishment, or foundation, where solo practitioners and two-man partnerships provide care in dispersed facilities under the aegis of a common plan organization.

National Health Planning and Resources Development Act of 1974 (Public Law 93-641). This is the latest in a series of bills that are predicated on the assumption that the medical industry is a utility in need of regulation. It virtually replaces the earlier areawide planning legislation. The act calls for 200 Health Systems Agencies to do the following:

- Gather and analyze health resources data.
- Establish health system plans (HSPs).
- Provide annual implementation plans (AIPs).
- Coordinate PSRO activity.
- Approve applications for federal funds.
- Assist states with certificate-of-need applications.
- Recommend programs to states for health care facilities development.

State Legislation

1. Legislation complying with the federal program has been enacted in most states.
2. Legislation enacted in all states permits professional service corporations for physicians. Indirectly, it encourages group practice.

IRS Regulations

Legislation in 1971 and subsequent tax regulations allow physicians in professional service corporations tax free deductions amounting to 25% or more of earnings for pension and profit sharing, virtually obsoleting the provisions of the earlier Keogh Act. Last year, Keogh was liberalized but not enough to replace some of the more lucrative professional service corporation pension plans.

BLUEPRINT FOR THE FUTURE

In addition to past and pending legislation, guidelines have been issued on how to develop health maintenance organizations. These guidelines together with legislation can be fashioned into a flexible blueprint, or model, on which to build health care establishments. The blueprint is largely acceptable to most of the power centers and largely in accord with provisions in pending legislation. It is sufficiently flexible to accommodate limited pluralistic approaches in developing new care centers.

Certain key features of the blueprint have not been determined, such as how the new system will be financed. There are various versions of how to finance the new system. Other than financing differences, there is much agreement on what the system should be.

Objectives of the Blueprint

Consensus among the power centers is that the new medical system should achieve the following objectives:

1. Provide each person with one place of access for comprehensive medical care.
2. Enlarge preventive care.
3. Provide a prepayment option.
4. Make care ultimately available to all.
5. Check the rising cost of care.

The blueprint also calls for a nationwide system of health maintenance centers, a universal payment system, and a system of government controls.

Government Controls

Like others, the medical industry is subject to many government controls which help form the overall blueprint.

Federal Controls

1. HEW regulates food and drugs by legislation.
2. It regulates clinical laboratories in interstate trade by license.
3. It administers Medicare treatment and payments through fiscal intermediaries.
4. It administers Medicaid through state agencies.
5. It administers Hill-Burton funds through state Hill-Burton agencies.
6. It sometimes regulates prices, fees, and wages through OPC.
7. It regulates planning and the administration of funds through the National Advisory Council and the Community Health Service Division of Public Health Service.

State Controls

1. Each state has a public health department that regulates environmental conditions, food, sanitation, inoculations, and other factors affecting health.
2. Each state licenses medical practitioners and institutions.
3. Each state regulates all medical associations incorporated within its borders.
4. Each state regulates planning at its own level by comprehensive health planning councils (A-agencies)— now being revised under the new National Health Planning Act.

Local Controls

1. Local regions such as counties and incorporated cities often excercise public health controls like the states.
2. They issue building permits.
3. They regulate planning at the local level by planning agencies (B-agencies)— now being revised under the new National Health Planning Act.

The blueprint of the future also includes the regulations of comprehensive health planning agencies. Recent legislation enlarges their part in funding new projects and controlling operations.

Comprehensive Health Planning

Under the blueprint, the national health planning system will be expanded. It will plan where health centers will be created and will distribute government funds for planning, development, and start-up operations. In fact, this is already being done. An estimated $400 million has been spent through the system to create hundreds of neighborhood health centers.

Federal Planning System

HEW is administering federal funds. It issues the ground rules, negotiates contracts, and approves grants for planning, developing, and operating community health centers. Technical guidance and liaison are provided in twelve regional offices throughout the country. Under the Bureau of Health Planning and Resources Development, HEW administers areawide planning at the state and local levels.

State Planning Systems

State health planing agencies, the A-agencies in process of revision under the Health Planning Act of 1974, must be consulted before a grant may be attained. In addition, state Hill-Burton agencies must approve loan guarantees made by FHA. But most important in the blueprint, the state agencies are responsible for issuing certificates-of-need.

The certificate-of-need is much like a liquor license — without one a proposed health center is likely to be thwarted. In fact, an HMO without a certificate-of-need is not an HMO at all. Through the certificate, the state planning agencies are exercising influence over where medicine will be practiced and who practices it.

Local Planning Systems

Local health planning agencies, the B-agencies in process of revision under the Health Planning Act of 1974, advise A-agencies on approving applications for funds and certificates-of-need. Through this advisory function, they also influence the development of medical centers.

Fiscal Blueprint

While it is still unresolved how the national medical bill will be paid — whether by government or a combination of government and private sources — certain features are agreed upon by most of the power sources:

1. Everyone should have access to essential care.
2. Comprehensive prepayment plans should be available to everyone.
3. Some control over utilization may be exercised by means of deductibles, copayment features, and nuisance fees for certain services.
4. Incentives for cost reduction, such as income sharing by providers, may be included.
5. Control over fees and costs should be adopted.

Capitation is a favored concept among the planners. According to this method, a health care center is paid a fixed sum yearly for the care of each one enrolled. Out of this stream of income, the center will provide the health needs of enrollees. Funds left over are shared by the provider members of the center.

Another favored concept is PSRO, which designates a whole range of provisions for seeing that quality care is given and that the public gets its money's worth. PSRO, now applied only to Medicare and Medicaid practice, is being readied for application across the board in the event that NHI is adopted.

Many of the health care plans call for capitation and PSRO. These two features are a part of the general blueprint. As legislation is adopted and complemented, the details of capitation and PSRO will be worked out. Right now the field is still open for innovation within this conceptual framework.

Comprehensive Health Care Organizations

The primary part of the blueprint deals with comprehensive health care organizations (CHOs). In 1970, HEW projected creation of 1,700 of these by 1975 to handle the health needs of 40,000,000 people. That amounts to around 25,000 people per center and gives some idea of the anticipated size planned.

Earlier projections had 90% of the population enrolled in health care centers by 1980. Assuming the date has been pushed ahead to 1985, this could mean 200 million people enrolled by then. If the mean size is still 25,000, the number of centers needed to accommodate the 200 million people would be 8,000.

Makeup of Health Care Establishments

CHOs differ primarily from other organizations and practices in one fundamental way. They give well-care in addition to sick-care. Their objective is to keep people well, to prevent them from getting sick, and when they become sick, to have them get well. In contrast, other health organizations, while giving some attention to preventive care, are more oriented to caring for the sick and less to keeping people well.

While the difference in the two kinds of organizations is largely one of emphasis — and therefore subject to debate — distinct differences show up in practice. A CHO enrolls patients and takes responsibility, though usually limited, to keep them well. The health of CHO patients is monitored by primary care physicians who give general care and arrange for special care when needed. As opposed to conventional medical practice, where the physician assumes responsibility for each illness as it comes along, the CHO gives continuous care under contract for a period of time. In fact, most CHOs charge a flat annual fee for care which enrollees pay regardless of how much they receive. They pay for well-care by the year rather than sick-care by the piece.

There are, of course, fee-for-service practitioners who give well-care. They watch patients carefully, encourage periodic visits, and prescribe checkups to detect incipient problems. Although many administer superior well-care, they do not formally take responsibility for giving such well-care. And in many cases, especially with new patients, or when physicians are busy, care is limited to the crisis kind.

CHOs are generally organized to give well-care. They specialize in patient education, inoculations, periodic checkups and other ways of providing such care inexpensively.

It is difficult to find a complete definition of a CHO since there are several kinds of well-care organizations. Kaiser Permanente is one type, Ross-Loos another, and Healthcare Association of Puget Sound a third. The HMO Act defines an HMO; but an HMO is just one of the many kinds of CHOs. In fact, the Kaiser Health Organization, the apparent model for the HMO Act, still does not qualify as an HMO under existing regulations.

CHO Provisions

Although you can't find a definition of a comprehensive health care organization, if you read the literature, you can abstract the essential components.

Here is one that fits about 95% of the concepts that are being touted. Notice the key words in italics.

A comprehensive health care establishment in an *association* providing a *comprehensive health care package* to *enrollees* for an *annual fee* under a *health care plan.*

Association. An association must include: (1) a health plan administrative function; (2) primary care physicians; (3) specialty providers; (4) a support services function; (5) adequate facilities; and (6) adequate financing. An association may also include: (1) a fiscal intermediary; (2) reinsurance arrangements; and (3) investors. It must serve a specified community and provide comprehensive health care. Organizationally, an association may be set up as a single entity or as a consortium of providers, tied together by contract, in accordance with an adopted medical plan. If it is an HMO, it must: (1) be a nonprofit organization; (2) have a certificate-of-need; and (3) have a community-oriented board of directors with consumer representation.

Comprehensive Care Package. The care package offered must include: (1) primary medical care including well-care; (2) specialty care, including essential surgery, inpatient care, and essential therapy; (3) emergency care; and (4) preventive care, including patient education, periodic checkups, inoculations, and well-baby care. The package may also include dental care and prescription drugs.

Enrollees. Eligibility for enrollment must include all who wish to enroll within each community served. Enrollees may be individuals living in the community; inhabitants of neighboring communities, or members of special groups such as unions, industrial plants, schools, Medicare, Medicaid, and others.

Enrollment may be limited to the care capability of a center by explicit, nondiscriminatory, published regulations. In brief, there can be no choosing of healthy patients over sick ones, or one race or creed over another, etc. The ground rules for selection should be sufficiently obvious to preclude charges of discrimination. This does not exclude group classifications for payment purposes, provided that no group is exploited in the process.

Annual Fee. The annual fee charged can include: (1) a fee for the basic service package; (2) optional fees for add-ons; (3) deductible provisions; and (4) copayment provisions. The annual fee can also be (1) adjusted to meet costs of care including fee-for-service charges of physicians; (2) paid directly to a CHO or paid to a fiscal intermediary that reimburses a CHO either on a capitation basis, fee-for-service basis, or both; (3) tailored to special groups such as Medicare enrollees; and (4) augmented by insurance.

Health Care Plan. The health care plan must spell out its objectives, the relationships among participants, the service systems and procedures used, and its financial systems and procedures. It must prescribe that its primary care physicians commit most of their working time to the plan; that they devote the time so allocated to treatment of enrollees; that they share in the process of a plan in accordance with a suitable formula, e.g., if they are reimbursed on a fee-for-service basis, any surplus or deficit should be allocated among them; and that other providers either join a plan on the basis prescribed for primary care physicians or enter into agreement to provide services on demand for a fee. The health care plan may also include provisions for the part-time services of member providers, mixing private patient practice with enrolled practice, and for continuing physician-patient relationships as private patients join the plan.

Thus, the comprehensive health care establishment as a concept is flexible enough for a variety of organizations.

A comprehensive health care establishment is comprised of a *health plan administrative function, primary care physicians,* services of *specialty care providers,* a *support services function, adequate facilities,* and it requires *adequate financing.*

Health Plan Administrative Function. The health plan administrative function can be an integral part of a CHO or a separate organization that contracts with the other participating groups involved. At a minimum, it must be responsible for:

1. Policy governing the overall establishment.
2. Enforcement of policy, including peer review.
3. Formulation of the health care plan.
4. Relationships with enrollees and providers.
5. Marketing of enrollee policies.
6. Procurement of medical services.
7. Fiscal management.

Primary Care Physicians. Primary care physicians must handle a patient's primary health needs, which include:

- Consultation, examination, diagnosis, general treatment.
- Initial emergency care.
- Preventive care.
- Referral for specialty care.
- Follow-up care.

Finally, primary care physicians of a CHO must join its medical plan as employees or as contract providers. Together with other providers who elect to do so, they must be members of the plan, providing services and sharing revenues.

As contract providers, they may organize in one of several ways: (1) as individual practitioners; (2) partners; (3) corporations; or (4) any combination of the three. Regardless of how they join, members may practice as a team in closed-panel facilities or as individuals in open-panel arrangements — or solo practice facilities — referring patients to others as necessary for specialty care.

Specialty Care Providers. Specialty care providers must be available to furnish services in the health care package, including: (1) office care of a specialist; (2) short-term and extended hospital care; (3) essential surgery and surgical support; (4) obstetrical deliveries; and (5) essential therapy. These providers may be either member providers who are employed or under special contract, or associate providers under contract to serve as required.

Support Services Function. The support services function must provide administrative support related to policy formulation, planning, contract administration, marketing, indoctrination of enrollees, purchase of provider services, and peer review.

It may also provide services pertaining to scheduling of care, booking, billing, bookkeeping, medical recordkeeping, drug distribution, facility operation and maintenance, supply, routine physical examinations, fiscal operations, transportation, communication, procurement, home nursing, diagnostic x-ray and clinical laboratory and data processing.

The support services function may be incorporated into the establishment as an integral part or as an independent agency serving the center under contract. As an independent agency, it can be: (1) a nonprofit corporation; (2) a profit corporation; (3) a division of a parent corporation or other association; or (4) a proprietary enterprise.

Adequate Facilities. Facilities must include: (1) sufficient space for the office practice of member providers, plan operations, and the support service functions; and (2) sufficient equipment to support these functions, including ambulance vehicles, emergency equipment, communications systems, and business equipment.

They may also include space and equipment for nonmember providers including inpatient facilities. The facilities should be: (1) conveniently located; (2) sufficiently integrated for efficient group action; (3) logically arranged; (4) ample for good operation, including sufficient parking space and patient waiting facilities; and (5) expandable. They may be owned or leased. New facilities and/or existing ones may be included for offices of solo practitioners who join the plan.

The configuration may consist of one facility, multiple facilities, or a central facility with satellites. Under the HMO program, two basic arrangements are permissible: (1) closed-panel facilities where physician groups practice together; and (2) open-panel facilities where they practice alone or in two-man partnerships.

Adequate Financing. Adequate funding must be available. Once a center is underway, it should generate sufficient revenues to meet expenses and provide for expansion. The critical need is for funds in the following phases of establishment: preliminary planning, development planning, facilities acquisition and construction, and start-up operations.

Preliminary planning involves designing a general plan for an establishment and testing it to see whether it will work. HEW has been giving grants of $25,000 to $50,000 for this kind of planning in the HMO program.

Development planning involves working out details to get started, including service packages, contracts for enrollees, providers and others, pre-enrollment recruitment, assay of enrollee health needs, systems and procedures specifications, building plans, financial plans, legal opinions, and precontract agreements with collaborating groups. HEW is giving grants of $100,000 to $200,000 for this effort in the HMO program.

Facilities acquisition and construction involves purchase and/or rental of land, buildings, and equipment including renovations and leasehold improvements. A center for 20,000 enrollees, if purchased in its entirety, would cost about $1,500,000 excluding inpatient facilities and around $6,000,000 if such facilities were included.

Start-up includes the operations from the day doors open to the public until the center breaks even. Funds are needed to meet deficits incurred during this period. Depending upon the medical plan adopted and community conditions, start-up funds can range from $100,000 to $4,000,000 or more per center. HEW is giving operating grants of several millions of dollars to HMOs for start-up.

Funds for creating a center may be obtained from the following sources:

- HEW grants for planning, development, and start-up.
- Public donations.
- Provider subscriptions.
- Private loans.

- Equity capital for the general services operation.
- Purchase leaseback arrangements.
- HUD grants for outpatient facilities and diagnostic equipment.

Loans on facilities and built-in equipment are eligible for a 90% guarantee under FHA provisions. Facilities and equipment may also be rented, reducing the amount of initial funding needed.

Optional Participants in CHOs

Optional participants of a health care establishment are:
- A fiscal intermediary.
- An insurer.
- A financial company.

Fiscal Intermediary

A fiscal intermediary, generally an insurance company, can share some of the marketing and fiscal burdens of an establishment. It can develop enrollee service plans, market them, collect premiums, and remit payments to the CHO. The intermediary can also share in the shortages and surpluses each year by establishing and maintaining an operating reserve fund.

Intermediaries and premiums are regulated by insurance laws of the states. Capitation fees can be adjusted as needed to meet expenses of CHOs, within rate guidelines prescribed for medical providers.

Insurer

An insurer that may also perform the intermediary function is prescribed for centers with less than 30,000 enrollees. The insurer may provide coverage for catastrophic cases where the medical cost of a patient exceeds several thousand dollars in one year. Also, the insurer can provide cash to meet expenses in a bad year.

Capital Company

A financial company can supply much of the funding for the health care establishment. It can: (1) purchase and lease back facilities and equipment; (2) provide working capital; (3) make building loans; and (4) provide profit-sharing and retirement programs for physicians and employees.

The financial company may be: (1) a commmercial bank; (2) an insurance company; (3) a small business investment company; (4) an investment bank; or (5) a private trust.

Optional Organization

The analysis shows that the components of a comprehensive health care organization are many and varied. While the blueprint specifically states what is essential, it allows flexibility. A variety of physical and organizational configurations is also possible.

Two contrasting types of organization possible under HMO legislation are shown in Figures 2-1 and 2-2.

In Figure 2-1, the CHO embraces all of the components. Physicians are hired and paid a salary. The board of trustees makes policy which is implemented by a management team headed by an administrator. The complex includes virtually all of the capabilities needed to render a complete health care package and relies upon associate providers to a minimal extent.

Figure 2-2 shows a consortium of organizationally independent groups. A plan administration unit creates the medical care plan and the contractual framework that ties the other units together. It gives

FIGURE 2-1

An Integrated Configuration

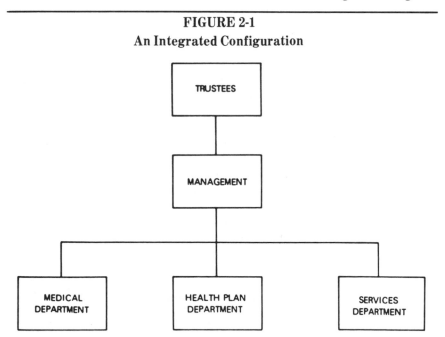

FIGURE 2-2
A Federated Configuration

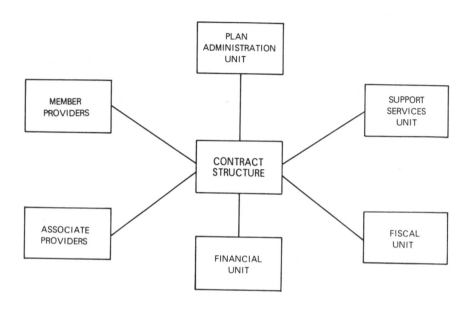

the overall guidance, acquires services and sees that enrolles get proper care. Each of the other groups does its part in accordance with the
medical plan. Physicians in this arrangement maintain their legal
status as self-employers, partners, or members of professional service
corporations. Other components, such as the services unit, can earn a
profit on services rendered and thereby attract private investors.

The organization described in Figure 2-1 is closely integrated; the
one in Figure 2-2 is more flexible. Each has its place, and there are
variations in between.

The blueprint for a comprehensive health care center is too broad
for an HMO at the present time. However, it is similar to the HMO
prescription, and, as the HMO prescription is broadened, it could conform with it.

BLUEPRINT IN ACTION

Although the blueprint for CHOs has been evolving for about 50
years, it took on most of its present form in the past decade. Six to

eight million people are already enrolled in medical centers that fit the general model.

Kaiser-Permanente

The most cited CHO is the Kaiser-Permanente Plan. Pushed by Henry Kaiser personally in the early 1950s, it has grown to serve over 2,000,000 enrollees. The operation is apparently very successful, and its earnings, computed on a profit-basis, have been compared favorably with Fortune 500 corporations.

While little factual information is available about how much it cost in investment dollars to support Kaiser's current growth, the sum appears to be quite large, as high as $1.0 billion or more.

The Kaiser operation was created to provide health services for the Kaiser Construction Company. After it caught the fancy of Henry Kaiser, it was expanded throughout California. Recently, it has branched out to other areas, such as Denver and Cleveland, where it has acquired extensive care facilities. The centers are relatively self-sufficient. They have nearly all essential medical resources, including inpatient facilities, surgeons, and other medical specialists.

Kaiser offers health care primarily to industry/labor groups on a family basis for a prepaid annual fee. Essential health care is included in the package. Preventive care is a highly stressed feature, but it is reported that only a small fraction of those eligible take prescribed periodic examinations.

The doctors at Kaiser are employees—at least they start that way—on salaries reported at around $35,000 to $50,000 annually. After two years of service, physicians can become quasi-partners, which simply means they share in operating surpluses distributed as bonuses.

Health care at Kaiser for a family of four costs $80 per month. This amounts to around $250 per person per year or about 60% of the national average for the kinds of services rendered. There is a small charge for an office visit, as well as copayments for extended inpatient care and other controls over utilization.

The lower cost of care at Kaiser has been explained in a number of ways:

- The enrolled group is relatively young and healthy. It includes industrial people in the prime of life with few elderly people. This could account for more than one-half of the difference in cost.
- Hospital bed days per person are reported to be 60% of the na-

tional average. This accounts for much of the remaining difference in cost.
- Reduced care, lower physician incomes, or greater efficiency in care practices may account for the reduced difference.

The lower rate of hospital utilization is explained by several factors: (1) the relatively low age of the enrollees; (2) Kaiser hospitals are not used for routine tests and diagnoses that can be performed in ambulatory facilities; and (3) certain operations such as tonsillectomy, appendectomy, and hysterectomy are performed less frequently per capita among the Kaiser groups.

Health Insurance Plan of Greater New York (HIP)

The second largest prepaid health care establishment in the country is HIP, operating in New York City and Long Island. This organization has been in existence for more than 30 years. It was originally created to provide medical care for the employees of New York City and has expanded to serve the general public.

HIP has expanded to a reported enrollment of approximately 800,000 people. It works closely with thirty physician centers consisting of approximately 1,100 physicians. It is an insurance company that markets medical coverage to the public and hires the services of the medical care centers. In some ways, it is like a super HMO: it sets the objectives, creates the medical plan, buys and sells services, and acts as financial intermediary and its own insurer.

Oddly enough the HIP medical package includes almost all essential services except inpatient care. It will currently obtain hospital beds for enrolles but expects them to have Blue Cross or other coverage to pay for it. This practice is in the process of being changed to include inpatient care in the basic package.

The HIP package includes office visits, surgery, care provided by specialists, maternity (excluding delivery), well-baby care, physical examinations, essential therapy, injection drugs, visiting nurse, and ambulance services. For these services, a family of three or more pays approximately $350 per year. Extended benefits, such as anesthesia in a hospital, emergency medical care, prescription drugs, private duty nursing, and medical health care can be covered by optional add-ons to the basic charge.

While HIP stresses preventive care, there is evidence that the turn out for periodic examinations is not large. Apparently, primary physicians do not push the periodic physical examination because of the work load that might be generated. Nevertheless, HIP operates, or is associated with, one of the most modern physical examination centers in the country and a large clinical laboratory which serves its physicians.

Finally, HIP is exploring the hospital business, having recently participated in constructing a 500 bed center in Queens, New York, to serve some of the borough's 200,000 HIP enrollees.

SUCCESS OR FAILURE

Judging from press releases and other information about comprehensive healthcare establishments, they appear to be successful. Former Secretary of Health Richardson, in his well publicized White Paper of 1970, stated:

> A variety of research studies and investigations have contrasted the cost of healthcare under HMOs with that of traditional practice. They all tend to the same conclusion: That HMOs lower the total health care costs of families and individuals, and that their premiums cover a greater percentage of total costs.

Group Health Association of America, a spokesman for the large HMOs, says in a brochure:

> Federal Employees Health Benefits Program data illustrate the lower rate of hospital utilization for members of prepaid group practices. During the year January to December 1968, for active employees, the indemnity insurance utilization figure was 1080 days per 1000; for group health plan members the figure was only 560 days per 1000. For dependents, the figures were: indemnity, 765 days per 1000; group practice, 305 days per 1000. The age—adjusted figures for all covered persons were: indemnity, 934 days per 1000; group practice, 429 days per 1000.
>
> The figures for non-maternity, in hospital surgical procedures for the high option Blue Shield and group practice plans are just as striking. The Blue Shield tonsillectomy rate was more than 250% higher than that of group practice plans. For female surgery the figures were: Blue Shield, 9.2 procedures per 1000; group plans, 4.8 procedures per 1000. The rates for all surgical procedures were: Blue Shield, 75 per 1000; group plans, 34 per 1000.

Another study compared 1965 health expenditures for the Kaiser-Permanente Medical Care Program of Northern California to the State of California as a whole. Annual age-adjusted per-capita hospital costs were: Kaiser-Permanente $34.30; State of California $56.06. The per-capita costs of physicians services were: Kaiser-Permanente $44.32; State of California $67.00 to $88.00 The total per-capita expenses were: Kaiser-Permanente $81.83; State of California $131.82 to $152.82.

While impressive on the surface, these figures are subject to attack. Closely analyzed, they reveal a bias on the part of those trying to prove the superiority of comprehensive care practice. One doesn't find the AMA publishing them as frequently as the proponents of HMOs.

But most important, there is no guarantee that putting off or avoiding medical treatment is good in the long run. In a system where the incentive is to keep costs down, it is possible that needed care may not be administered when necessary but rather postponed. The figure 4.8 surgical procedures per 1000, instead of 9.2 per 1000, could be looked upon as evidence of gross neglect rather than the elimination of blatant butchery. Since members of the medical profession are hardly likely to be guilty of either practice, it would seem that either the statistics are wrong or there is much judgment latitude in deciding whether or not to perform a medical procedure. The latter supposition would appear to be the more likely.

On the matter of financial success or failure, the question is somewhat clearer. In spite of grants and preferential treatment, many health care establishments, especially HMOs, fail. They are expensive to get started and often don't hold together. The reason is that the federal formula for HMOs contains provisions that could be ruinous in the long run. Under the federal concept, implemented by seminars, HEW has encouraged HMO sponsors to invade neighborhoods, set up practice, and recruit enrollees. Great emphasis has been given to marketing — doorbell ringing, mail campaigns, and visits to industry to get mass enrollment. This method of instituting an HMO is unusually costly, and of questionable ethics, as the recruitment programs often take patients away from nonsubsidized practitioners already in neighborhoods invaded.

An alternative approach would be to consolidate existing practices in the neighborhood. Not only would the ethics be better but development and start-up costs would be considerably less. This approach, however, might violate some cherished tenets of government planners — tenents that have apparently contributed to HMO failures — such as practitioners should be employees, which is anathema to many practitioners, and that health care establishments should be reimbursed for services on a capitation rather than a fee-for-service basis. The employee issue is dear to bureaucratic people. Since they are on salary, they think everyone else should be. Moreover, employee practitioners can be controlled better than contract practitioners.

Most physicians, however, have a different view. They see themselves as professionals providing services under agreements in which they play an equal, if not dominant role, in the relationships.

Capitation is a favorite theme among government people because many medical economists erroneously believe that it is the only method of payment that will hold down health care costs. They correctly antiticpate that a fixed sum to keep people well will discourage overuse of medical care, as opposed to the present system that encourages overuse. However, what they underemphasize is physician fear of capitation, the financial risks involved in it, and the fact that it takes a large health care center to absorb this risk.

Indeed, there is an economic conflict between the size of centers that are likely to thrive in the initial stages of group care and the size needed to handle the caprices of capitation. Big enough for capitation is often too big for getting started.

Despite several handicaps, some health care enterprises manage to flourish. What is their secret? Most, if not all, of those that succeed do so because of an extenuating circumstance — generally an unusual demand for health care services that brings purchasers and suppliers together in a cooperative effort. New HMOs, which are apparently successful, have been sponsored, financed, and subsidized by insurance companies, unions, investors, and industrial companies that expect to buy their services. Some of those that have user backing and appear to be successfully launched are the Columbia Medical Plan, the Harvard Community Health Plan, the Genessee Valley Health Association, and the Maricopa Foundation for Medical Care.

Furthermore, health care centers seem to do better in closed communities than in bedroom communities. In a closed community, where people work and live, chances of getting a combined user-and-provider sponsorship is greater than it is where inhabitants go off to work in distant communities.

The blueprint discussed in this chapter is derived from documents issued on the evolving medical system including guidelines issued by HEW and incorporated in pending legislation. Although it is remarkably specific, it also gives reasonable latitude and conforms with documents written by diverse groups of people.

Most important, the blueprint has sufficient latitude for practitioners to create the kind of practices they want. They don't have to accept the cherished tasks of government planners. In fact, they can select those features that are professionally desirable and fall within the parameters of the public blueprint.

Chapter 3
Strategy for Participation

How do you participate in the changing system of health care? There is no single answer. It depends upon who you are and your individual situation. The prime movers of the industry are 360,000 physicians and 120,000 dentists. The present system is built on them just as the new one will also be built on them; and they naturally will take part in shaping it. There are 100,000 medical and dental students, who will form the backbone of the new medical industry as well as hundreds of thousands of other medical providers such as opticians, therapists, parameds, nurses, and others.

Sixty thousand pharmacists, and the major drug companies, will also be interested in the evolving system, since most drugs will be distributed through health care centers. Many centers already have drug dispensaries, and some economize significantly by using generic rather than trade names. Also, economy is gained by mail order practices. HIP, for example, furnishes enrollees all prescribed drugs for $15 per year by mail order, less than one-half the national per capita cost.

Thousands of clinical laboratories which perform around 4.5 billion tests annually will also be affected. With emphasis on preventive medicine, they will double their volume in a few years. It is likely that some laboratories will join the doctors to form health centers.

Approximately 8,000 hospitals, 8,500 clinics, and 15,000 nursing homes will participate. Hospitals can join physicians to form health centers or become associate providers with a group of centers. A large hospital with several hundred beds can become a service hub supporting six or more satellite care centers operated by groups of its physician staff.

Unions, industrial groups, schools, and government agencies are eligible for creating care centers. Many may be created by county medical societies, which number in the thousands. Foundations and insurance companies, such as Blue Cross, Prudential, and Connecticut General are collaborating in the development of health centers.

Local communities are natural sponsors of care centers, since most centers will serve a community and will require significant local participation. Some 5,000 or more town, city, and county governments could sponsor care centers, not to mention public-spirited citizen groups.

Besides the obvious providers and sponsors, other groups that will be affected include government workers, contractors and equipment suppliers. A special role might be filled by service corporations, providing the support services of centers. Up to 10,000 service units will be required to furnish $15 to $20 billion of support services annually. These services can be furnished by profit-making corporations. Corporations specializing in facilities management, administrative services, and other services already operate units in health care centers.

Insurance companies will be called upon to perform fiscal intermediary and insurance roles. As people enroll in prepaid plans, they will phase out of conventional plans. Up to three billion dollars of annual fees will be at stake, which will involve the jobs of several hundred thousand insurance employees.

It is reported that more than $40 billion of capital will be required to create health care centers — capital for planning, development, acquisition of facilities, and operations. Government will probably provide 20% of the capital; the remainder will come from private sources. Loan guaranties and other incentives will be used to attract investors. Venture capitalists, banks, insurance companies, and SBICs will find opportunities.

As centers are established, they will need retirement plans, which could conceivably generate up to $10 billion annually for the investment channels of banks, insurance companies, and mutual funds.

Finally, consultants will be needed. The job of planning, developing, and creating a health center is largely a one-time effort requiring specialists. Management consultants will make feasibility studies, formulate objectives, develop implementation programs, and make organization plans. Industrial and business engineers will create systems; contractors will do facilities planning, and lawyers will draft contracts and secure certificates, permits, and licenses. All told, thousands of professionals will help reconstruct the industry.

PHYSICIAN STRATEGY

Physicians will play the principal role in restructuring the industry. Since they largely run the existing system, it is inconceivable that it can be built without their consent, cooperation, and leadership. The community of physicians has misgivings about restructuring the medical industry. While no one has taken a conclusive poll recently, it is not difficult to find doctors who are opposed to the blueprint. One could bet safely that a majority would vote against much of the blueprint for change. The American Medical Association endorses a universal health insurance plan but is careful not to put an unqualified stamp on HMOs.

Individual practitioners appearing at congressional hearings have opposed various congressional plans. They cite some compelling factors against the blueprint:

- The preventive care proposed is not worth its cost.
- It would increase the load of an already overloaded industry. Giving everyone just one annual physical would require the full-time services of nearly one-half of the primary care physicians and would add about $15 billion to the annual cost of medicine. medicine.
- Group practice has not proved more effective than solo practice.
- **The existing system is more flexible than the one proposed.**
- Changeover will be too costly.
- Extending government controls will add costly red tape, reduce incentives among medical workers, and introduce unnecessary restrictions.
- Incentives to reduce care by capitation will encourage patient neglect.
- Encouraging well-care will bring out the hypochondriacs who will swamp the system.

Although the arguments are good, they are being offered too late. Even though a majority of physicians oppose the blueprint, it has apparently gone too far to be stopped.

Strategy of Dissent

One strategy is to sit it out and hope that the status quo will remain—an unlikely possibility. It is not likely that the power centers will give up easily. The opinion makers have already convinced the public that a new medical system is needed, and politicians are going to give the people what they want. Even in the face of opposition, government controls many of the health care purse strings and under universal insurance will control more of them. Through a system of incentiveness — "rewards" for those who go along and "punishment" for those who balk — the government will almost certainly exercise enough influence to get physicians into the new system. Those who drag anchor could find their practices dwindling away as outsiders invade their communities. The one who sits by and watches could find himself on the outside looking in with little say over the kind of practice that will prevail in his community.

The strategy of wait-and-see, however, is not all bad; it could be a good one for some practitioners. Those who are five years or less away from retirement have little to fear because the movement is not going fast enough to overtake them. The superspecialist who is in great demand certainly can afford to wait and see what develops, since he may never find it necessary to change his method of operating.

Others who want to dissent have three choices: (1) quietly quit practice; (2) quit practice while making a big issue of it; and (3) continue practice and fight the changes taking place. Competent dissent is needed. While it will not likely stop the underlying trends of the industry, it could slow them down, and could even obviate features that might be disastrous in the future. The American Medical Association, for example, by insisting upon pluralistic methods of practice, is providing needed opposition to those who would put all physicians in HMOs. Lawsuits by AMA and others are aimed at undesirable features in PSRO, the favoritism given to HMOs, and planning legislation that treats the medical industry like a utility.

A Physicians Bill of Rights, published in 1975 by *Physician's Management*, set forth below, presents more grist for the dissent mill:

Physicians' Bill of Rights

1. Physicians are entitled to fair treatment.
2. They are also entitled to due process of law.
3. They are entitled to freedom in the pursuit of their livelihood as long as the public is properly served.
4. They are entitled as a professional group to self-regulation.
5. They are entitled to be free of government regulation except where self-regulation is inadequate.

6. Government regulation should be limited to what the doctor does, not how he does it.

7. Physicians are entitled to challenge each government regulation and to offer suitable alternatives.

8. While under appeal, a regulation should be suspended.

9. The burden of proving the need for a regulation should rest with the government.

The dissenting physicians can contribute to the opposition movement by developing constructive suggestions, writing articles for **publicaton and for congressmen, medical societies, and lobbyists,** making speeches, appearing before legislative groups, and contributing to political action committees.

A program of dissent against the Big Brother aspects of medical legislation in *Physician's Management* suggested the following tactics:

Suggested List of Legislative Goals

1. Stop nationalization of health care.

2. Amend the HMO act to extend special privileges to all practices.

3. Limit areawide planning authority to government financed facilities.

4. Make all practice facilities, including all hospitals, eligible for **Federal Housing Administration loan guarantees and for tax-ex**empt municipal bonds.

5. Remove all bias in the law against proprietary practice.

6. Remove all controls in the law predicated on the assumption that the medical industry is a utility.

7. Amend all laws regulating medicine to provide an effective appeal mechanism, with the burden of proof for the need of specific **regulations resting with the government.**

8. Restore competition to halt abnormal price increases.

In a program of dissent, physicians can try to preserve these *endangered options:*

1. The option to organize in pluralistic ways.

2. The option of patients to choose conventional practice as well as prepaid practice.

3. The option to mix conventional with prepaid practice.

4. The option to be reimbursed on a fee-for-service basis.

5. The option to preserve doctor-patient relationships.

6. Retention of tax and other favorable advantages in legislation covering professional service corporations.

7. The option to install pluralistic control procedures.

Dissenting physicians should direct their lobbying efforts at the states as well as the federal government. In implementing federal legislation, states can tighten up on provisions and make the blueprint totally undesirable. Conceivably, they could put all doctors on salary, regulate their hours and rates of pay, and install controls that would be both demeaning and crippling. Constant surveillance and active lobbying may be necessary to prevent this.

Strategy of Participation

Most medical practitioners have to go along with the system whether they like it or not. Participation doesn't preclude dissent, however. A strategy of participation is needed in either case.

The easiest way to participate in the current scene is to jump right into it. As the old saying goes: If you can't beat them, join them — a strategy that is fine for those who have no sizable stake in an existing practice, and no compunction about getting into a group or other institutional practice. It is a strategy that most medical students will embrace and one that some successful practitioners will find desirable. But joining the movement may not be as simple as it seems, especially for the discriminating practitioner. There are the knotty problems of selecting a group or institution to join and of getting accepted.

The strategy of a young intern may be simple, particularly if he or she is gifted. He will probably go where he can get the best training, regardless of where. But sooner or later he too will be faced with decisions on where and with whom to practice, and his decisions could be crucial to his career.

Those looking for long-term connections in the evolving system should understand the underlying movements that shape it. They should familiarize themselves with different kinds of care establishments so that they can make the first critical choice: the kind of establishment they want to join. They might consider the following kinds of practice:

- Public Health Service
- Hospital staff member
- Industrial medicine
- Health care establishment

- Conventional group — multispecialty
- Conventional group — single specialty
- Two-man partnership
- Solo practice

The list is ordered to correspond to the emotional needs of practitioners. At the top, job incumbents find the following conditions: (1) work structured by others; (2) negligible job risk; (3) limited challenge (generally); (4) regular working hours; and (5) limited compensation. At the bottom of the list, the following conditions prevail: (1) self-structured work; (2) considerable job risk; (3) high challenge; (4) unpredictable, long working hours; and (5) compensation dependent on ability. In the middle, conditions vary between the two extremes in accordance with position.

In view of underlying changes taking place, physicians who lean toward solo practice might wisely consider group practice instead. While solo practice is likely to continue indefinitely, it is on the wane. Ten years from now, if present trends continue, only the superspecialists will be able to survive in two-man partnerships and solo practice. Those who like solo practice and see themselves as future superspecialists should elect it. The others should get into group practice.

Those who decide on group practice will find another challenge in selecting among a range of practice types. They can join health care establishments that provide comprehensive care or conventional care groups that give limited care. Within each one of these major categories, there are further choices:

Patients treated:	Well-to-do? Middle class? Poor? Mixed?
Location:	East Coast, West Coast, Midwest, etc.
Neighborhood:	Ghetto? Inner city? Suburban? Rural?
Compensation type:	Salary? Salary and bonus? Fee-for-service?
Restrictions:	Many? Some? Very few
Support services:	Many? Moderate number? Few?
Fringe benefits:	Many? Moderate number? Few?

For most, finding the exact type of practice desired will probably be somewhat of a compromise between the ideal and what is available. So it is important that practitioners seeking long-term career connections start early in their quests to see what is available. Using proper discretion, especially if they are already employed, they should gather as much information as possible about what is available by interviews and letters to organizations that look promising. Sources for opportunities include: U.S. employment service, the Civil Service Commission, private placement agencies, university employment services, medical societies, and trade publications.

The American Medical Association has a master list of clinics in the U.S.; Interstudy of Minneapolis keeps an inventory of HMOs; and the American Association of Foundations for Medical Care of Stockton has an inventory of foundations. Almost all large cities have mailing houses with lists of group practices by states.

As soon as possible, those seeking career connections should establish criteria for the kind of care center desired. The criteria should be broad enough to include further narrowing in accordance with specific opportunities. Questions should be raised about the group's reputation, how progressive they are, their long-term prospects, and their treatment of new physicians. Most important for each applicant is whether he can get along with the other members of the group. The final test is whether the group wants the applicant. Finding a good career opportunity is difficult, but a good strategy can facilitate the process.

For those who already have a practice, the strategy of participation must include a decision on what to do with the practice. Those who pick up stakes and go elsewhere have to get rid of old practices. Those who stay where they are may have to close their practices but more likely will have an opportunity to merge them with others.

Practitioners who are established in a given neighborhood and wish to remain there need a special strategy to meet new challenges. Solo practitioners, two-man partnerships, multispecialty groups giving limited care, and those single specialty groups that cannot stand on their own in the long run will face growing pressure to organize in groups and offer comprehensive care. If they resist, many will be threatened by organizations that do provide such care.

While it is somewhat unusual to discuss medical practice in business terms, it is a fact of life that medical practitioners, like others in the economic arena, have markets for their services. Many of those markets have been built up over the years through painstaking practice. Today many of them are threatened by new kinds of practice — HMOs and other health care establishments. Some of the competing establishments are given favored treatment — grants, financing guarantees, revenue funding, and other favors in order to make them flourish. Moreover, the certificate-of-need procedure sponsored by the federal government and administered by the states could lock out conventional practices as officials promote new practices in their place.

How should threatened practitioners face up to this situation? What kind of strategy should they employ? They should join forces with neighboring physicians and create associations to advance the medical services of their communities. Those who are already in clinics will be one step ahead in this process. The associations can be loosely organized at first. Through a process of evolution, slowly or rapidly as the situation may dictate, they should progressively integrate themselves as opportunities for cooperation and joint ventures materialize. At the onset, the associations should examine the medical needs and resources of their communities, determine how needs can best be met, keep abreast of all threats to existing practice, get to know public officials and influential citizens, and establish community health care objectives.

At a later stage, the associations, especially if they are threatened, can draw up plans for creating health care establishments, file them with government planning councils, and apply for certificates-of-need. In this way, they will at least participate in formulating the care centers of their communities and possibly block others from taking away their markets.

In the meantime, the dissenting physicians can keep the pressure on lobbyists. While they may not be able to reverse the tide, they can keep matters from getting worse. Resourceful physicians can still make a lemonade out of a lemon. As long as the flexible provisions of the blueprint remain, dissenting physicians can create and file fairly respectable plans. It is important, therefore, to keep this flexibility.

HOSPITAL STRATEGY

Aside from doctors, hospitals will be most affected by the evolving system of medical care. About 50% of all care is rendered directly and indirectly through hospitals. With emphasis on preventive medicine, the new system is designed to reduce need for inpatient care. Moreover, hospitals could be relegated to the role of associate providers, entirely dependent upon health care establishments for their livelihood—especially if health care establishments take on responsibility for managing all the care of their enrollees.

Looking at the situation a bit more optimistically from the hospital's point of view, there is an option under the blueprint for hospitals to sponsor health care centers, create them, join with them in a variety of ways, and to take other roles in the evolving system. The question arises: What should a hospital do under these circumstances? It depends of course, on the hospital — its size, relationship to the community, and other factors.

Size is one of the most important factors governing the strategy of a hospital. A large hospital with fifty or more doctors would find it difficult, if not impossible, to create a single health care enterprise. It would have to line up most of its medical staff and bring them into one organization, an almost impossible task. Furthermore, a large hospital would have to enroll 50,000 or more patient members, and unless most were from the surrounding community, the logistics of its operations would be unwieldy.

The small hospitals with twenty-five doctors or less could be an ideal nucleus for a comprehensive health center, particularly in a closed community where the doctors are relatively compatible with one another. Further, if the community happened to be dominated by one or two industrial companies cooperative about the idea of health care establishment, the chances of successfully organizing a center would be even better.

A large prosperous hospital can afford to sit by and watch the creation of health care establishments. As centers are set up in neighboring communities, such a hospital can offer services to each center as an associate provider and can charge prearranged fees. If it signs up enough service contracts, it can continue to prosper. Some large hospitals may desire a more active role. They may be feeling the pinch of expanding costs and contracting budgets and may not want to diminish the demand for services. Such hospitals may have some eager young men who are looking for new challenges. These hospitals can encourage their medical staff to create health care centers. The hospital, conceivably, could be the supporting center of multiple health care satellites. In addition to providing the necessary inpatient facilities and services, a hospital could provide support services and thereby expand activities.

Another option for the large hospital is to become a member provider of a health care establishment. In this capacity, the hospital would share capitation gains and losses. While this might involve risk, it has the compensating advantage of giving the hospital first-hand experience in the health care business. A logical approach would be to join other groups either as a member or associate provider, and later consolidate them into a large health care establishment. While it may be impracticable to create a CHO out of a large hospital at the start, this gradual approach could accomplish the job in the long run.

A small hospital has many choices. It can follow the courses prescribed for a large hospital or go ahead and create a health care center with its medical staff. How should a hospital administrator proceed if he wishes to take an active role? The following steps are recommended:

- Become familiar with the blueprint for remaking the medical industry.
- Learn as much as possible about health care centers.
- Contact the regional HEW office and tell them what you are considering.
- Ask for their advice; receive their mailing lists, and place yourself on federal mailing lists.
- Become familiar with the state health department and make the acquaintance of officials who can help you.
- Clip news items from newspapers and magazines on the new medical system.
- Familiarize the board of directors, the medical staff and others about health care centers.
- Explore the hospital's role in the evolving system of health care.
- Determine what role the hospital should play.
- Obtain authorization to proceed, then go ahead.

If the decision is to create a health care center, the hospital should take the steps prescribed for physicians, namely to create an association and file a plan. In this way it will become eligible for federal aid and, at the same time, stake out a claim on the territory.

Mercer Hospital in Trenton is one of the first in New Jersey to support an HMO. Working with twenty-nine physicians, it is helping to develop an HMO for residents of Trenton and surrounding communities. The HMO, known as Mercer Regional Group, has received grants from the federal government. New Jersey Blue Cross is working closely with the Mercer Group, marketing its policies and serving as financial intermediary. According to news articles, proposed care at the center will not come cheaply. It will cost $75 per person per year more than basic Blue Cross/Blue Shield coverage. However, according to Dr. Milton Epstein, head of the group, the center will give nearly complete medical care for the increased amount.

Another enterprising group is Hunterdon Medical Center in Flemington, New Jersey. It is a hospital of 195 beds with office facilities for thirty-seven physicians. Like Mercer, the hospital and medical staff have gotten together to create an HMO. It has received two federal grants already, a planning grant for $48,000 and a development grant for $100,000. The center will serve a rural area and is expected to move slowly as a result.

Almost all of the new HMOs — numbering several hundred — work closely with hospitals. Some are sponsored by hospitals, others are joint ventures with hospitals, and many use hospitals as a base of support.

Bellwethers in this movement are the investor-owned hospitals. They include some of the largest corporations operating hospital chains in America. These, accounting for more than 5% of the beds in the country, are gearing up to provide comprehensive care and support services to health care establishments.

INSURANCE COMPANY STRATEGY

Insurance companies, particularly the Blues, have a large stake in the system of medical care. They are virtually faced with either a new lease on life or the prospect of fading away.

How can they meet the crisis? One strategy is to wait for the verdict. If Kennedy legislation is passed, they might decide to phase out of the business entirely. The crucial question is really what to do in the meantime. Insurance companies that wait are likely to find themselves behind the parade, while those that go ahead may waste their efforts.

The proper strategy appears to be going ahead and gaining experience with health care centers. At the present time, it looks as if insurance companies will play a large role in the new industry. Even if Kennedy-type legislation passes, there will be a need for catastrophic insurance and for administrative and fiscal services which insurance companies will provide. Furthermore, the cost of going ahead on a limited basis is small to gain the advantages of getting started early.

Insurance companies that are interested in going ahead should create task forces for exploring opportunities. They should: (1) become familiar with the blueprint for change; (2) keep up to date; (3) explore the potential market for services that the company can provide; (4) draw up tentative plans for participation; and (5) joint venture with others in the creation of prototype health care centers.

As insurance companies become involved, they will find that their new role differs significantly from the old one in several ways. They will become community oriented rather than industry oriented, since health care centers are largely community setups. A center serves a given community, gets most of its enrollees from it, and most of its providers. Insurance companies will need to get used to these facts. In working with CHOs, they will work with communities much as they worked with industry, establishing community and even provider rates much as they now do with industrial or experience rates.

One feature that insurance companies might provide at the start is a series of riders to its basic policies to conform with the prepayment needs of health care centers. Riders should cover catastrophic illness, preventive care, office visits and other services needed to make conventional prepaid coverage equivalent to comprehensive coverage.

Some insurance companies are already joint venturing experimental centers. Connecticut General is working closely with Columbia, Maryland, to develop an HMO that will serve the entire community. It is reported that the company not only participates in current fiscal operations but also provided start-up capital. Prudential Insurance, which is offering to finance health centers, suggested in a recent brochure that it can do better than the government. Many of the Blues are also getting into the act. The Rochester Blues have joined with community organizations to develop several HMOs for Rochester and Monroe County in New York, aided by a $300,000 HEW grant.

Insurance Companies that wish to get started on a joint venture with communities should prepare or acquire a library of flexible planning documents to cover typical situations. They should construct a service line around these documents and a program to merchandise it. Hospitals, medical associations, individual doctors, and officials at local communities should be solicited. Out of this effort, an insurance company can select capable joint venturers, and start its file of prospects for the future.

SERVICE COMPANY STRATEGY

The potential role for service companies is extensive. Projected medical centers will require management and administrative talent that can be furnished by these companies. In addition, they can furnish many medical support services. Potential services of $15 billion (in 1976 dollars) by 1981 make it attractive to large companies skilled in rendering service to the public.

Like insurance companies, service companies should plan on creating local units that will serve as associate providers in forthcoming health care centers. A service company could conceivably have 500 or more local units, organized nationally and regionally in a single company. Hospital service corporations, equipment rental companies, hotel corporations and others have much of the knowhow needed to service contemplated medical centers. These companies get into the business in much the same way as the insurance companies.

Once they decide to go ahead, they should develop sufficient documentation to construct a variety of centers, solicit the prime movers in progressive communities, and experiment with model centers.

FINANCIAL COMPANY STRATEGY

Financial groups will have one of the largest stakes in the industry. With $40 billion of capital needed, many opportunities for providing capital will be available. The strategy for most financial groups is likely to be one of waiting for things to develop, since those who need capital will seek the financial groups, not the other way around. However, there are special advantages for those that take the initiative. Not only will they capture the best opportunities, but they will find new sources of investable capital in centers they create. A health care enterprise needing $3 million in initial financing, for example, is likely to generate $500,000 in investable funds yearly — in interest, repayments, and pension funds.

The financial groups that want to take an active role will have to seek suitable partners for coventuring: an insurance company, service corporation, or possibly a consulting firm that has plans for sponsoring health centers. As a preliminary step, financial companies should draw up plans for financing real estate and buildings and equipment under various conditions. They might also develop plans for furnishing working capital. Finally, they might prepare a variety of retirement plans and other investment plans for the participants of the centers.

CONSULTING FIRMS

Consulting firms will play a large part in the evolving system. They will provide much of the documentation needed. However, only those who adopt an aggressive role will play a large part in the development. It will be advantageous for them to draw up essential documentation for their specialties: management engineers will design organization and system components; construction engineers will create alternative design approaches; and so forth. With this documentation, they should seek opportunities to venture with others (physicians, hospitals, and insurance companies).

OTHER GROUPS

Other groups that could take an active role include companies, unions, government agencies, schools and local communities. A company can create a health center for its employees much as Henry Kaiser did orginally. It can cooperate with the local community in setting up a center, or pick up the bill for insurance riders. A union can accomplish the same thing by bargaining with a company. Most government agencies can underwrite a comprehensive health plan for their employees under civil service provisions. The decision to take an active role depends upon how much these groups value modern health care and its alternatives. Important considerations are the savings by reducing absenteeism and improving employee effectiveness, the goodwill generated, and the fact that health services can be provided to employees tax-free.

Universities and preparatory schools, where students are away from home for most of the year, should carefully consider creating in-house health centers. These institutions have a responsibility for the care of students; they also exercise this responsibility at a critical time when the student should be forming good health habits and establishing a baseline for monitoring health in the future. With a virtually captive group of enrollees, the large school could establish an effective health maintenance center with little risk.

The public officials of local communities are probably the most logical supporters for health care centers because a center is largely a community affair. The mayor of a city can do more than almost anyone else to get one started. He can generate local interest, provide seed capital, and enlist medical practitioners.

PAYERS OF HEALTH CARE

Last, but not least, are the payers of health care who also need a strategy for participating in the evolving system. In a free economy, those who pay generally get what they want in the long run. Health care providers will ultimately conform to what payers want. The strategy of the payers will make a difference in how fast the medical system evolves.

In order to analyze the role of payers in the medical system, the overall U.S. health care bill can be conveniently divided into two parts. Twenty percent of it, about $25 billion annually, is for long-term hospital care, care of military dependents, veterans' care, research, public construction, and public health services. The other 80%, about $105 billion, goes for conventional care of the civilian population. The 20% part is paid by government; the 80%, by government, industry, and individuals. It is the 80% that ultimately controls the medical industry. At present, this part is almost equally divided among government, private industry, and self-paying individuals.

Much of the self-pay is for deductibles and copayment of insurance policies. It is really part of the general insurance program, an augmentation of the industry and government shares of the total medical bill. In addition, both government and private shares of the payment have been growing while the self-pay share has been shrinking. Before long the ratios will change from 33:33:33 to 40:40:20, as self-pay is reduced to cover only the deductibles and copayments associated with a universal insurance program. Indeed, the present payment profile is so close to what it would be under NHI, there is not likely to be the drastic change that people expect when NHI is passed.

Today there are two large classes of payers for medical care: government and private industry. Through wishes of their constituents, they will determine what the health care system will be in the future. As dissatisfaction with health care grows, both government and industry are showing concern. Many people want comprehensive health care and can't get it. Everyone seems to be disturbed by the skyrocketing costs. Company benefits directors are skeptically viewing health insurance costs as the cost of health care jumps one-half of a percentage point on the GNP scale each year.

Both government and industry apparently need a strategy to get what they want. Government's strategy is well known. It is attempting to hold down prices while maintaining quality of care by controls, such as PSRO. Occasionally, it has resorted to price fixing, but only in times of severe inflation. Most significant has been the program to create a national system of HMOs to take care of all patients who want care through them as well as Medicare and Medicaid patients.

One faction of government wants a national health insurance bill that would replace private industry payments for health care by government payments. This would, in effect, make one payer for all health care, the federal government; and it follows that under such conditions the government could dictate the kind of care it wants. Government, of course, would get the money to pay for care by higher social security taxes that in turn would come out of what private industry now pays for health insurance.

To a large extent, government strategy has bogged down. Many congressmen are not willing to put the health care system under control of one customer. The HMO part of the strategy has also bogged down because of unrealistic requirements that keep most care centers from becoming HMOs. PSRO, area planning and other programs are experiencing difficulties because of red tape and what appears to be constitutional over-reach.

But even if government strategy worked, it would have severe limitations. Industry and private citizens still control most of the conventional health care buying power. What industry does still makes a vast difference in how the medical economy shapes up.

Up until now industry has gone along with the inflationary insurance system that plays such a prominent part in the medical industry.Outside of a few companies that are experimenting with health care systems for their employees, companies pay the annually increasing cost of health insurance and pass it on to customers through price increases. There is nothing to check overuse in the system, except the deductibles and copayments which are weak deterrents at best. Physicians generally do not assume responsibility for health maintenance, except on a piece by piece, or episodic basis; and they are not held responsible for cost of care. In short, the present system discourages responsibility for cost. Moreover, physicians acting individually are not in a position to change the insurance system. They haven't the means or the power to do so.

The press and some public officials have lashed out at insurance carriers for failing to police medical costs, but carriers too have little control over the system. About all they can do is encourage development of health maintenance centers, which they do to a limited extent. Meanwhile, the system remains unchanged. Of all those involved, industry appears to have the best opportunity to break the chain. Like government, the other big payer, it can demand the option of health maintenance for its employees. It can ask insurance companies to certify both physicians and clinics that will provide comprehensive health care.

Moreover, in taking this approach, industry can avoid some of the mistakes of the HMO program. Health care packages can be made competitive with conventional coverage. Health care establishments can be created to attract practitioners rather than repel them. For example, if physicians want to be paid on a fee-for-service basis, there is no disadvantage in doing so provided responsibility for the care costs of beneficiaries are pinned down to providers so that a provider-rating system can be established. Under a provider-rating system, high cost providers will be weeded out unless they justify their higher costs in some way.

In a system where care and cost responsibility are pinned down, industry can develop measuring sticks for cost of care. Employees electing high cost providers can be charged a premium to compensate for the higher costs. In this way, the cost control features envisioned in HMO legislation can come into play without distasteful features and cost-push factors in the existing program.

With such an opportunity, major companies and industries might well consider changing their present strategy of waiting passively to one of actively exploiting a private industry form of dual choice. If such a strategy is adopted, it could well develop into a general movement. The benefits executives, representing the payers of health care, could establish and work up health care programs through community councils with representation from the medical industry, the insurance industry, and government. Such a movement could be in the interest of the free enterprise system. In recent years, real earnings of industrial employees have declined partly because of rising medical costs. This in turn has raised the question as to the efficacy of free enterprise. Any improvement in the health care system will, therefore, strengthen free enterprise. It would also benefit several groups. The movement would assist insurance carriers to set up dual option plans, and it would aid medical practitioners to develop the medical industry and possibly help them avoid nationalization.

Finally, government, the other big payer, might alter its strategy somewhat to encourage a private movement. Some of the things government could do to promote both its own strategy and a private one are:

- Adopt a partnership policy with industry (the other big payer of medical care) to attain an effective health maintenance program.
- Modify HMO specifications to eliminate present undesirable features not consonant with objectives of cost-controlled health maintenance.
- Eliminate favorite treatment extended to government approved HMOs.
- Reduce restrictive regulations on development of health care establishments such as the certificate-of-need requirements of the states.
- Revise liability laws to protect medical practitioners from extra liability they will take on in giving health maintenance and well-care to enrollees.
- Adopt income tax regulations that limit industry deductions for medical care to per capita amounts that conform with reasonable yardsticks under cost-controlled programs.

The strategies of participants are not only implementing the public blueprint, but they are interacting with it to reshape it. The present and future strategy will determine the new configurations that evolve and will retard or accelerate underlying movements changing the medical industry. These strategies are clearly pointing toward the development of group practice.

Group practice is becoming the building block of the emerging medical system. It is through group practice that industrialization, the constructive aspects of federalization, and the comprehensive care movement exert their major impact on the nation's health care system. For these reasons, strategy for participation in the emerging system of medical care is largely centered in the development of group practice. Group practice, in turn, is the primary objective of strategies that have evolved in the changing medical system.

Chapter 4
The Pros and Cons of Group Practice

For some practitioners, the handwriting is on the wall. They must get into group practice in order to save their practices. Consider this recent occurrence in California: a sound truck comes into a suburban neighborhood and announces the availability of a utopian health plan—a new HMO has been created that will keep patients well, a place where anyone can go for care and where the doors are open around the clock. Care will be given for any kind of disorder, but more than that, the place will "assume" the responsibility of keeping enrollees well. Further, the new center will cost most enrollees very little. Calcare and Medicare will pick up the bill for the indigent and aged, and employers will pick up much of the bill for others— so it is claimed.

Whose patients are they taking? Obviously, they are taking the patients of other physicians in the neighborhood, from solo practitioners including those who have built up practices over many years. Moreover, the new clinic is being financed and encouraged by government, by taxes levied on existing practices. It is not very fair, possibly unconstitutional, but nevertheless a fact of life, and a situation that is likely to get worse for many years. Furthermore, if the existing solo practitioners wait long enough, they may be shut out altogether. By the time they get around to creating a competitive clinic, they may find they cannot do so. For example, they may find it necessary to get a certificate-of-need. But with the new HMO firmly entrenched, the government may find another clinic unnecessary.

Thus, it is better for practitioners to form a group practice now rather than wait until others "steal" their territory. Many of those who see the handwriting on the wall are swamped by regulation, litigation and growing social demands that have virtually disrupted the medical industry. In addition to PSRO and other legislation, the courts have been tough on the medical industry and have made the practice of

71

medicine hazardous, not just to the careless practitioner, but to the good one as well.

Also, as patient insurance coverage and other third party payment grows, there is more paperwork for physicians which becomes difficult and perplexing for those busy with patients. These changes are too strenuous for many solo practitioners, who in addition to being physicians, must acquire some expertise in law, accounting, and business administration. It is not simply that they will lose patients if they don't become multitalented, or get sued, but they will run the risk of engaging in "criminal practice." For these reasons, they feel a need to band together, to jointly seek the services of legal and business experts, and to get the moral and intellectual support of peers facing the same problems.

The reasons for creating group practices are not only defensive. There are also positive reasons for forming or joining a group. The chief one is to improve the care of patients. Before the current upheaval in medical practice and the big push by the government for HMOs, about 30% of the nation's practicing office physicians went into group practice, creating thousands of clinics. The single specialty clinics were in large part created to raise the level of treatment for special disease, while the multispecialty clinics were created to widen the spectrum of patient care along the one-stop principle. Some of the single specialty clinics have grown to become large nationally known institutions such as the Menninger Clinic for psychiatric care, Krile Institute for bone surgery, and Sloane-Kettering for the treatment of cancer. Some of the multispecialty centers have grown to become giant institutions such as the Kaiser Health Organization, the largest health establishment in the United States.

Although groups don't always provide better care than solo practitioners, they have the opportunity to do so by pooling patients and resources. Certain aspects of preventive care, such as periodic examinations, laboratory tests, inoculations for epidemics and childhood diseases, and the maintenance of patient records can be handled more effectively — both in terms of quality and cost — for large numbers of patients rather than for small numbers. The pooling of resources and larger patient loads in a clinic make it economical to use sophisticated systems of care not in the reach of solo practitioners, such as automated laboratories for health examinations and clinical chemistry, computer systems for maintaining health records and making medical analysis, and emergency life-saving equipment.

Sharing economic resources is another reason why practitioners set up a group practice. Often the sharing progresses gradually. As a Cleveland physician put it:

> Our clinic really got started fifteen years ago when Dr. Smith and I decided to jointly rent an office downtown. At first we shared a nurse-receptionist and an after-hours answering service. Then we began to relieve one another on urgent cases at vacation time. Concurrently, we kept one another informed on important developments in the medical field. Several years later a third associate joined us, and we expanded our sharing to include an outside bookkeeper and accountant. Then eight years ago we took a big jump. Together with a fourth practitioner we built a medical center in the suburbs that would house eight practitioners. The four of us set up practice under a single shingle, took possession of the building as a partnership, and rented the remaining space to four other physicians. Now the eight of us are considering putting it all together to form a comprehensive health care clinic.

Finally, many practitioners are attracted to group practice for financial benefits. The doctors from Cleveland, for example, invested in a facility to get tax deductions on interest and depreciation. Later, they set up a professional service corporation to gain more tax advantages. Groups also take some of the pressure off physicians who can work fewer hours than solo practitioners. Moreover, physicians in a group can earn more money than solo practitioners by superior systematizing.

While opportunities abound in the growth of group practice, there are advantages and disadvantages which should be carefully considered. Patients who enroll in a group practice will find advantages and disadvantages compared to solo practice; medical practitioners will also find pros and cons; and suppliers will find drawbacks as well as bonanzas.

PATIENT ADVANTAGES AND DISADVANTAGES

Some of the advantages for patients who join a comprehensive health care organization are: (1) one place to go for all medical care; (2) a flat fee, or modified flat fee for all care; (3) continuously available care; (4) emergency care; (5) fewer referrals to other care centers; (6) better equipped and supported physicians; and (7) preventive care. The disadvantages may involve (1) a change of one's personal physician or dentist; (2) less personalized care; (3) more care administered by physician assistants; (4) reduced choice in selection of attending physician; and (5) slightly higher cost of care.

Some of the disadvantages depend upon the particular clinic selected, the philosophy of its practitioners and circumstances of the patient. For example, if a patient's physician and dentist are members of a group in a facility across the street from him, he obviously will not have to travel for care. Treatment by physician assistants in cases where a physician is not required could be superior and is certainly less costly than it would be if administered by a physician, in which case it would be an advantage rather than a disadvantage. Continuity with one's own personal physician will depend largely upon how a specific clinic is run.

The outstanding advantage will be the benefits of preventive care where such care is administered. While the merits of preventive care are highly controversial, some aspects such as inoculations and health education are unquestionably beneficial. The economy and practicality of giving everyone in the nation a periodic physical examination — as envisioned by health planners — are debatable. Many claim that it would take up most of the time of primary care physicians and raise the cost of care more than 25%, at least initially, before preventive care programs reduce the need for curative care. Nevertheless, in the long run, preventive care should reduce unnecessary disease and the cost of medical treatment.

PRACTITIONER ADVANTAGES AND DISADVANTAGES

A 55-year-old physcian who joined a sixteen-member group practice in a bedroom community in New Jersey sums up his five-year experience this way:

> My life changed entirely when I joined the group. Until then, I had been a rugged individualist, a typical solo practitioner, responsible for the care of 1,500 patients, on call day and night, feeling guilty every time I avoided a patient call, and never fully at ease even on vacation. After two of my classmates died of heart attacks, I decided to join a group. Now the pressure is not nearly so great. My patients get better care; and believe it or not, I can handle more patients with somewhat shorter hours.

This attitude and other similar opinions testify to the advantage of group membership for physicians and other practitioners. They enjoy better facilities, a closer association with peers, peer support in adversity and greater productivity. Group membership often provides superior support services while giving practitioners more leisure time, higher earnings, and less pressure and exposure to malpractice charges. The financial advantages involve increased tax shelters as well as estate building opportunities.

Advantages cited are obviously dependent upon the particular clinic joined. A well-run clinic can give better care, treat more patients per physician day, and yield more income to practitioners than a solo practice; while a poorly run clinic will give less care, treat fewer patients, and afford less income than a solo practice. The solo practitioner, therefore, runs a certain risk when he joins a group. However, the superior effectiveness of group practice in general is borne out not only by logic but by most studies on the subject.

While professional practitioners often tend to overlook the remunerative aspects of medical practice, success of group practice in the long run and its ultimate dominance over solo practice may well depend upon tax shelters and estate building opportunities. Government treats groups much better than individuals in this respect, and the difference could be the margin between a prosperous practice and a barren one. For example, in income tax practice, the IRS allows as tax deductible any expense that is made to advance the welfare of an organization as opposed to its single individuals, including so-called nontaxable fringe benefits such as food, lodging, life insurance, employee care, health insurance, convention expenses and education. Even tax deductions for education of the children of physicians in clinics are being claimed with support of reputable tax attorneys — apparently with some success. With most physicians in tax brackets around the 50% level for their last increments of income, nontaxable fringe benefits can make up a hefty part of their compensation — gains made by legitimate deductions from an otherwise staggering tax load. Diversion of funds into the pockets of physicians in this way, which is sizable in well-organized clinics, could make a considerable difference in the economic welfare of group practice professionals.

The major opportunities for tax avoidance are in investment programs. Here again, the advantages are weighted in favor of group practice over solo practice. Many physicians who own their own facilities and rent to others are taking advantage of accelerated depreciation and other arrangements that reduce their tax load. But most important are programs for retirement and estate building, made possible under a labyrinth of federal and state laws, that require professional guidance which is much too expensive for most solo practitioners.

Table 4-1 compares the estate building capability of two physicians starting at midcareer — one in solo practice without a formal retirement program, the other in a health care center with a full-fledged program.

TABLE 4-1
Estate Building Capability
1976 Dollars

Item	Solo Practitioner	Center Practitioner	Advantage Center Practitioner
Professional earnings	$1,100,000	$1,100,000	$ —
Capital gains and interest	489,000	880,000	391,000
Insurance receipts	200,000	200,000	—
Less premiums paid	(100,000)	(100,000)	—
GROSS INCOME	$1,689,000	$2,080,000	$391,000
Taxes	526,000	508,000	18,000
NET AFTER TAXES	$1,163,000	$1,572,000	$409,000

Assumptions: 20 years of practice followed by 20 years of retirement. Annual consumption rates: $22K for solo practitioner, $30K for center. Estate at Death: $283K for solo practitioner, $372K for center practitioner.

As indicated in the above table, which is based on a conservative set of assumptions, tax shelters recently provided by legislation make it possible for a particular practitioner to realize at least $400,000 more during his remaining career and retirement span than a solo practitioner without a plan. It is true that a solo practitioner can establish a retirement plan under Keogh, and at considerable risk a much more liberal one by creating a one-person professional service corporation. But he is better off in a group for the following reasons:

1.   A plan requires expensive professional help for its creation and continual monitoring, a cost almost prohibitive to the solo practitioner, but modest when shared in a group.

2.   Very lucrative plans, made possible by incorporating, are risky when applied to a corporation of one person, as the IRS specifies that incorporating for tax avoidance only — hard to disprove in a corporation of one — disqualifies tax exemptions.

3.   A plan must be actively monitored if not defended in the tax arena, which is another world for the typical solo practitioner.

4.   Many solo practitioners haven't gotten around to considering an adequate retirement plan for themselves, much less their employees, and many of them postpone the problem. Groups, on the other hand, can afford to delegate the problem to qualified professionals.

5.   Many solo practitioners who have set up plans have done so through part-time tax advisers, moonlighters, and others with questionable backup, getting in turn either modest Keogh plans or risky plans under the other more beneficial regulations.

There are also disadvantages of group membership which often involve (1) group entry and protocol requirements; (2) surrender of some independence; (3) shared misfortune with other members of the group; (4) decreased flexibility; (5) sharing authority; and (6) unwanted colleagues.

These disadvantages, however, vary, depending upon the situation. Some clinics require the surrender of almost all independence. HMOs, for example, often make employees out of practitioners, and in effect "supervise" them — a situation most physicians reject. However, physicians need not become employees of a clinic, unless the clinic mandates it. Depending on how the clinic is created, they may practice with almost the full independence of the solo practitioner. Some group practices have been created literally in accordance with the doctors' prescription, attaining for their practitioners all of the advantages of group practice while retaining many of the advantages of solo practice.

Chapter 5
Anatomy of Group Practice

The basic building block of the new system is the CHO, which could be replicated up to 10,000 times. Each CHO is a complex of operating systems that fits with others to form the overall industry. Supplementary building blocks are provider groups that serve two or more CHOs, such as corporations providing the support services, insurance companies providing fiscal services, hospitals providing inpatient care, and investors providing capital.

Like the cells of a human body, CHOs will make up much of the new medical economy. Each one will be part of it; and all combined will make up much of the whole. While units other than health care centers will exist, they will operate largely within the influence of CHOs. Thus, a composite picture of a CHO reflects in microcosm the evolving system of medical care.

CHOs often evolve from conventional group practice. The process is one that starts with a new practice that develops into a mature establishment. Some establishments skip early phases of development to become CHOs at the start. But even these encounter much of the typical experience in the slower evolution. Thus, group practice is pivotal if not crucial in the evolving system. It is the main arena of development—not just for CHOs that emerge from the process, but for budding CHOs as they mature, and for specialty care groups that serve them.

Since CHOs come out of simpler forms of group practice, the anatomy of group practice represents the full range of group establishments from simple primary forms to complex CHOs. Group practices are diversified. They range in size, complexity, services administered, scope of care, patient makeup and internal structure. As the saying goes, no two groups are alike—even HMOs differ from one another. Kaiser hardly resembles HIP, and HIP differs considerably from the Harvard Community Plan.

Nevertheless, they all have a common anatomical model. The wide spectrum arises from a combination of common components. A knowledge of the anatomy of group practice helps analysts understand the spectrum of group practice, how the group practice movement can be promoted, and how individual establishments can be developed.

A group practice in the broadest sense is a subsystem of the medical economy. It consists of the following major components: market, operating establishment and supply sources. The operating establishment is a bridge between its supply sources and market. Resources originate in centers of supply, and are acquired by the operating establishment where they are converted into medical services. The services are, in turn, distributed to patients who make up the market. The flow is a straight line of values, from sources to market, as follows:

SUPPLY SOURCES → ESTABLISHMENT → MARKET

Group practice anatomy covers the full span from sources to market. It is best understood, however, by starting at the end of the line and working backwards. The endpoint of a practice is its market, which largely determines how the rest of the practice is structured. Thus, market is the logical starting point in a discussion of group practice anatomy.

MARKET

The term market has not been used frequently in the medical industry until lately. Physicians used to set up practice in a neighborhood, and patients came until the physicians were fully occupied. There was no thought given to market. But as doctors practiced in groups, and groups grew in size, the need to maintain a sustained flow of revenues became serious. With the emergence of giant care centers, such as Kaiser and HIP, revenue continuity became critical, and medical people began to talk about markets. Today, when HEW gives seminars on HMOs, the emphasis is on how to market medical services.

The market of a health care enterprise consists of the *territory* it serves, the *patients* within it and their *demand for care*. In dollar terms, it is summarized annually by amount of revenues generated. Each care establishment that receives revenues has a market either all to itself or shares one with other providers. Its *territory* and *patients* may or may not be shared.

Territory

A territory, loosely defined, is the geographical area where a care enterprise seeks patients. Generally, it is a local community as most centers get patients from their neighborhoods. But this isn't always true, especially for large or unusual establishments. Some, because of their reputations, draw patients from all over the world. Others have branches in neighborhoods that are dispersed and not necessarily contiguous with one another.

Mainly, territory is the neighborhood, but it often is restricted to a small radius — sometimes just a part of a neighborhood, because patients are reluctant to travel far for care. With the exception of rural and underserved areas, patients are not likely to do so. In places with high population density, territories are considerably constricted, and there are often many providers whose territories overlap. In places of low population density, territories often stretch over several neighborhoods in wide areas where patients must travel a long distance whether they like it or not, because the community is not large enough to support a full-time physician. In such areas, care centers often have little or no competition.

Patient reluctance to travel not only limits size of territories but size of care centers, too. The larger the center, the larger the territory it needs; and even in dense communities, the large centers must draw patients from distant places to keep fully utilized. This logistical principle has kept care centers smaller than planners like, and will probably keep them small for some time to come. Health care establishments get around this limitation on size per center by creating centers in many neighborhoods.

Another limitation on size is population density. Where population is sparse and as a result territories are larger, there are likely to be many small centers, instead of a few large ones, thereby cutting down patient travel time. Federations of solo practitioners are suited to this kind of market because they have small, widely dispersed units.

Under the public blueprint, a CHO will have a territory, serve that territory, be identified with it, and to a degree, be bound by it. The blueprint may change on this point, but probably only slightly. Kennedy-type legislation calls for somewhat strict territorial jurisdiction, while some HEW officials talk about eliminating territorial restrictions altogether. It is difficult to see how Kennedy-type provisions can be enforced without introducing serious limitations. At the same time, the industry can't be regulated without some territorial restrictions. For example, issuing a certificate-of-need is strictly a territorial matter. Many other territorial controls could be required, such as community capitation rates, and measurements of health progress of a community.

Furthermore, a health care center must be geographically cohesive. It must draw largely upon local resources and serve local patients. In short, it is by nature a local affair oriented to a community, identified with it, and to a degree, bound by it.

There are latitudes that may be necessary in forthcoming regulations if the system is to work smoothly and competitively. First, while each center will have a territory, a territory should be allowed two or more centers for competitive purposes. Second, patients should be allowed to cross territorial boundaries to join a health maintenance center in another neighborhood. Third, providers should be allowed to cross territorial boundaries and serve centers in two or more territories. Fourth, facilities dispersed over two or more territories should be allowed. Fifth, two or more centers should be allowed to overlap in serving an area.

The blueprint is still relatively flexible on the matter of territory, although certificate-of-need laws are encroaching on territorial options. Also, as areawide planning legislation is implemented, it could be more restrictive than it is now. It is safe to assume, therefore, that there will be many legal battles, legislative amendments, regulations, and interpretations before territorial guidelines are finalized.

Patients

Patients, the most important part of a market, are classified according to:

Age:	Senior citizens
	Children
	Infants
	Others
Sex:	Male
	Female
Means:	Poor
	Middle class
	Well-to-do

Ethnic group:	White American
	Black
	Hispanic
	Other
Type of care received:	Conventional care
	Comprehensive care
Entry decision:	Self entry
	Referred entry
Payer or sponsor:	Medicaid
	Medicare
	Private insurance
	Self-pay
	Other
Entry status:	Enrollees
	Nonenrollees

The classifications are useful, especially for projecting health service demand. Senior citizens, for example, require three times the amount of care of young patients. Females of child-bearing age need more care than males in the same age group. The poor require up to twice the amount of care that others need. Patterns of care also vary among ethnic, age and sex groups.

A significant classification is *type of care given.* Patients receiving conventional care are handled differently than those under a comprehensive package. The entry decision varies. In general and multispecialty practices patients come of their own accords, while in single specialty centers they are referred by other practitioners.

Care packages and supporting operations depend upon who pays. Third party payers impose peculiar specifications for care, record keeping, fees charged, and billing and collecting for services. Also, considerable difference exists among payer groups in the time taken to pay bills.

Finally, some centers enroll patients for annual care; others do not, accepting them as they seek care with each episode of illness. Some centers have both kinds of patients, and therefore dispense treatment that differs considerably for each kind.

Under the public blueprint, patients in an HMO can be enrollees or nonenrollees. They may enroll in a center and for an annual fee get comprehensive health care; or they may continue as they do now, paying for individual services. Those who enroll are member patients; others who use a center or its physicians are nonmember patients.

The fees of HMOs are regulated by HEW and include incentives to curb unnecessary use of health services. For payment, members get a basic package of benefits, including some health education, checkups, emergency services, physician consultation, inpatient care and surgery. They may also receive drugs, dental care, psychiatric treatment or optional add-ons to basic premiums. Nonmember patients pay for services as received either by cash or insurance voucher.

A CHO is obligated to care for member patients on a continual basis and to see that nonmembers receive services paid for at each episode. The patient-doctor relationship of a nonmember is usually a private matter for which a center is not directly responsible. However, there is a provision in the HMO Act stating that physicians in HMOs must devote the majority of their working time to enrolled patients.

A center is morally obliged to enroll all residents in its territory — regardless of race, creed, color, or health condition — according to an orderly plan. It may enroll residents of other communities and treat transient patients. HMOs are required to have open enrollment once a year — a stipulation which will probably be rescinded.

Sources of patients, once taken for granted by the small clinic, are important to the large clinic and to those trying to become large. They include: residents of the neighborhood; referrals from other practitioners; transients; members of local industry; unions and schools; persons on Medicare and Medicaid; military dependents; civil service and other government employees; and members of religious and fraternal groups.

The list can conveniently be divided into two parts. The first three items are conventional sources that until recently required negligible market effort. The others are largely new sources that usually demand health maintenance programs for beneficiaries. Marketing approaches are being developed by HEW and others to capture patients from the latter sources; and a sizable effort has been mounted in parts of the country to actively recruit patients from them — including advertising and doorbell ringing that is offensive to much of the medical profession.

Patient groups often have service contracts tailored to their needs with special payment rates. Sponsors such as Social Security, representing Medicare enrollees, negotiate terms for their beneficiaries and pick up part or all of capitation payments.

Finally, patients interact with CHOs in other ways. They may have a voice on boards of trustees, which under HMO legislation is mandatory.

Demand for Care

Demand for care in a territory depends largely on patient mix and service available. A breakdown of health care distributed by patient category nationally shows that 25% are elderly, 15% are poor (excludes the elderly) and that other persons make up the bulk of 60%.

Excluding long-term institutions and federal facilities, per capita care annually in 1976 was approximately $500. In places that have more elderly and poor than their share per capita, the demand is higher; and the reverse is true in communities with relatively young and prosperous inhabitants. The basic demand for care is shaped by available services. In California, where comprehensive care is fairly abundant, more people want it. Metropolitan areas like New York City have many outpatient facilities which consequently are in high demand. On a national basis, demand for medical care (excluding long-term institutions and federal facilities) is shown in Table 5-1.

TABLE 5-1
Demand for Medical Care, 1976

	%
Hospital: inpatient	40
outpatient	5
Physician office[a]	25
Dental	8
Drugs[b]	6
Nursing home	5
Diagnostic radiology[b]	3
Clinical tests[b]	3
Prosthetics	3
Other	2

Notes:
[a]Includes surgery
[b]Excludes hospital share

The medical market of an individual center depends not only upon territories and persons served, but also upon services offered. Centers offering only office care are usually limited to 25% or less of the total market. Practitioners who further limit care to a specialty might have 1% or less of a market. However, the territories served by rare specialists are often larger in accordance with the scarcity of these specialists.

The practice of comprehensive care broadens the market of a center in a given territory. Health care centers operating under the one-stop principle could conceivably supply 100% of the medical market. Many centers are already providing most of the care demanded in their communities.

OPERATING ESTABLISHMENT

The operating establishment or internal makeup of a group practice is dependent in part upon the market it serves, its goals, and its limitations. Some facilities grow by setting their sights on market objectives that they try to achieve with available resources. Others set up the best possible practice and hope the public will beat its way to their doors. Many grow in a topsy-turvy fashion but in the long run are shaped by market forces and their own latent capabilities.

The internal structure of an establishment can be viewed from three useful vantage points. First, the establishment can be considered a collection of basic resources structured in a physical configuration. Second, it can be viewed as a set of operating units structured organically; and third, it can be viewed as a collection of systems structured sequentially.

Basic Resources

An operating establishment includes land, buildings, equipment, working capital, people, and other resources. Physical resources can be owned, rented, or purchased, as needed. Success depends on how well resources are combined into centers and systems of operation to meet market demands.

There is a fundamental trade-off between the acquisition of resources and the purchase of services that resources provide. Often the old saying applies: Why buy a cow when milk is so cheap? Instead of ambulances, the center buys ambulance service; instead of hiring maintenance people, the center buys maintenance; instead of a clinical lab, the center contracts for lab services. Just about every service can be purchased so that a trade-off can be made between buying capital resources and acquiring their services.

The resources of any one establishment depend, therefore, on the market it serves and how much it relies on external resources. Patterns exist relating resources of typical centers with their operating characteristics. A rough recipe of requirements for a fully self-reliant

CHO is listed:
- 1 primary care office practitioner per 1,800-2,000 enrollees.
- 2 specialty office practitioners, including dentists, per 2,000 enrollees.
- 3 hospital beds per 1,000 enrollees (after several years of preventive care).
- 1,000 square feet of floor space per bed.
- $40,000 worth of equipment per practitioner.
- $40,000 worth of equipment per bed.
- 3 support people per practitioner.
- 2.5 support people per bed.
- 8 parking spaces per practitioner.
- 4 parking spaces per bed.
- 1 acre of land per practitioner.
- 1 acre of land per bed.
- $150,000 capital investment per practitioner.
- $150,000 capital investment per bed.

According to this formula, a full-fledged CHO serving 50,000 enrollees would require the following:
- 25 primary care practitioners.
- 50 specialty practitioners.
- 150 hospital beds.
- 225,000 square feet of floor space.
- $9.0 million worth of equipment.
- 600 support people.
- 1,200 parking spaces.
- 22.5 acres of land.
- $33.8 million investment at original cost.

The blueprint for HMOs is fairly flexible regarding basic resources. An HMO can subcontract with a hospital or other care institution to take care of its enrollees. It can purchase the services of specialists as needed. It can also purchase the services of outside suppliers, which can be profit-making organizations. All that is required is the major time of sufficient primary care physicians and enough administrative talent to provide enrollees with comprehensive care either inhouse or in the facilities of subcontract providers.

Organic Structure

Less than a dozen sets or dimensions, each simple in itself, combine in a half dozen ways to make up the wide range of organic configurations found in group practice. A practice hangs together organically by its organizational structure and the physical structure of its facilities. Often, it is designated in terms of organizational units, like the Kaiser Organization, and its internal units are designated divisions, departments, and sections. Just as frequently, it is referred to in physical terms, terms like complex, center, unit, and branch. The elements of both kinds of structure have peculiarities that require separate treatment.

Organizational Structure

An organization structure is one organizational unit or several combined units. An organizational unit, in turn, is a group of people performing one or more related functions in accordance with a set of working agreements. A logical formula defining the organizational unit is: ORGANIZATIONAL UNIT = PEOPLE • AGREEMENT •FUNCTION(1...N)

Multi-unit organizations come in a variety of hierarchical structures as indicated in Figure 5-1.

FIGURE 5-1
Hierarchical Organization Structure

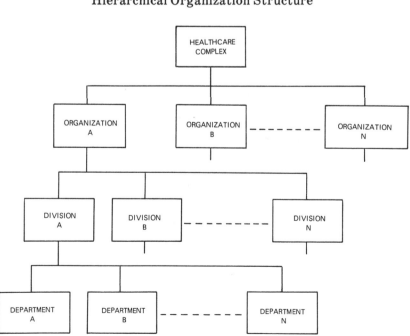

Three kinds of basic agreements hold an organization together: (1) those tying principals to principals; (2) those tying principals to employees; and (3) those tying principals to suppliers. Articles of organization, partnership arrangements, etc. tie principals together, and the structures they set up are often called *external or legal organizations,* largely because the agreements both require government endorsement and control many external relationships— particularly how the enterprise is taxed and publicly regulated. Employment agreements and subcontractor agreements for inhouse support, based on job structure, form the internal or operating organizational structure.

The agreements that tie principals together designate various legal types of organizations, such as proprietorships, partnerships, corporations (for profit or not), cooperatives, joint ventures or other associations.

Often a complex organization has one or more establishments, each with its own form of legal organization. The most common arrangement is the holding company, generally a corporation that owns corporations. There are also other combinations, such as an association of corporations or partnerships, and a nonprofit corporation holding profit corporations and the reverse. Almost all combinations are found in group practices.

Internal structuring is largely determined by the way functions are grouped together to form jobs and job structure. How each job in an enterprise is formed and how jobs are combined into sections, departments, divisions and entire organizations depends upon the size of each enterprise, geographical distribution of its parts, the care it administers, and available resources. The number of configurations is large and consequently there are few, if any, establishments that are alike in organization structure. Even within similar constraints of size and so forth, there are options on how to organize.

There is, however, a basic functional pattern common to health care establishments. Though the range of functions performed varies, especially between large and small centers, the establishments perform common functions that can be classified and described. For such purposes, it is convenient to consider a large establishment model, keeping in mind that a small or limited establishment many have less functional content than the generic model indicates.

A large and integrated health care establishment generally has three basic functional units: a health plan unit, a health care unit, and a service unit. These units are often subdivided as follows:

FIGURE 5-2
Division of a Complex

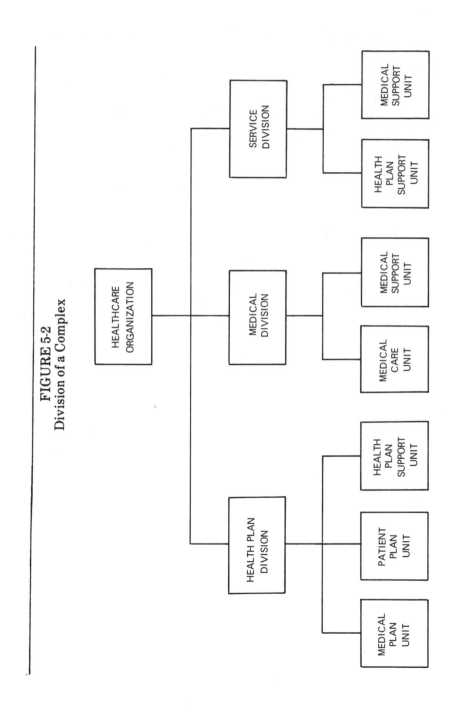

In a CHO, the health plan unit sets up and administers contracts that tie providers and enrollees together in an integrated system of health care. It often contains a subunit for providers, another for enrollees, and one for administrative support of the health plan unit. The basic function of the health plan unit is to buy care from health providers and furnish it to enrollees.

The health care unit administers health care services. It consists of primary care, specialty care, and inpatient units, as well as support units providing backup services closely allied to medical care.

The service unit supports the other units. It generally contains subunits and performs routine functions that can be done best off-line, or out of the mainstream of activities. While many services must be performed on-line, such as critical examination of patients, others, such as billing, bookkeeping and routine testing can be done either on-line or off-line in specializing units.

The internal structure of a CHO is largely determined by decisions on what functions should be performed in specialized service units. As centers grow in size, the number of functions that can be economically performed off-line grows. The volume of common services becomes large and opportunities for profitable specialization arise. Billing chores that keep a nurse busy part-time in a small center become large enough as the center grows to keep several billing clerks busy, and ultimately, large enough to require a computer section.

These growth opportunities for service specialization are tempered by the operating preferences of physicians. Some physicians will relinquish routine functions readily; others will not. For example, many doctors are willing to have their billing and bookkeeping done by a service unit, but only a few relinquish their booking of patients.

Some of the service units found in health care establishments are: facilities units; administrative service units; fiscal units; data processing units; clinical and dental laboratories; health testing laboratories; and consulting units.

Physical Structure

A physical unit or center is made up of one or more organizational units operating in facilities at a specific location. A logical formula defining a center is as follows:

CENTER = ORGANIZATION UNIT(1...N) • FACILITIES • LOCATION

Like organizational units, centers can be structured in hierarchical form as indicated in Figure 5-3.

FIGURE 5-3
Hierarchical Physical Structure

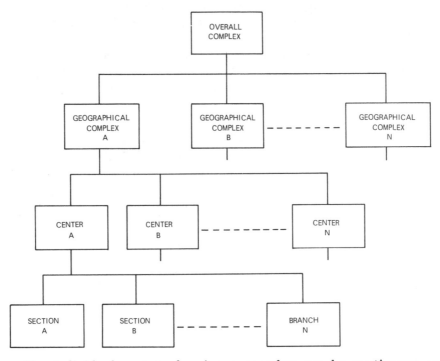

The individual centers forming a complex can be contiguous or separated from one another. This is also true of units making up a center. Almost any kind of combination is possible. The Kaiser Establishment is actually a collection of complexes, a supercomplex, spread out over several areas of the country. Many centers have branches that serve patients in their outlying areas.

The organizational and physical structures of each health care center intersect to form operating complexes. Just as there are medical plan organizations, medical practice organizations, and support service organizations, there are similar kinds of centers and complexes:

- MEDICAL PLAN CENTERS AND COMPLEXES.
- MEDICAL PRACTICE CENTERS AND COMPLEXES.
- SUPPORT SERVICE CENTERS AND COMPLEXES.

The physical configuration of a center relates to numerous factors: the market to be served; the systems of operation that provide health care services; the organizational units that make up the systems of operation; and the physical constrictions of territory and available resources. All must be taken into account—generally, in the order presented. The upshot is often a configuration that evolves out of many different compromises.

The public blueprint for establishing physical facilities is relatively liberal. However, it is complicated by areawide planning restrictions which could dictate the facilities that may be established.

Systems

The organic structure of a health care establishment is ultimately arranged to serve its operating systems. Just as an entire establishment can be viewed organically, it can also be viewed systemwise. From this vantage point, a health care enterprise is a complex of systems that accomodate the flow of services from medical providers to patients. Some of the systems are classified in the following outline:

I. Medical Care Systems
   A. Primary Medical Care
      1. Center Initiated Care
         a. Education
         b. Inoculations
         c. Periodic physicals
      2. Patient Initiated Care
         a. Office care
         b. Home care
         c. Outpatient care
   B. Specialty Medical Care
      1. Inpatient Care
      2. Surgery
      3. Physical Therapy
      4. Psychological Therapy
   C. Patient Logistics
   D. Medical Support Services
      1. Drug Dispensing
      2. Prosthetic Device Distribution
      3. Patient Examinations
      4. Chemical Lab Operations
      5. Radiology Lab Operations
   E. Transportation Systems
   F. Supply Systems

G. Facility Systems
H. Personnel Systems
II. Fiscal Systems
III. Operating and Technical Information Systems
    A. Patient and Treatment Information Systems
        1. Patient Data System
        2. Medical Procedures Selection System
        3. Drug Selection System
    B. Medical Technology
    C. Medical Procedures
    D. Patient Education Curricula
    E. Employee Education Curricula
IV. Administrative Information Systems
    A. Management Systems
        1. Policy
        2. Long Range Planning
        3. Short Range Planning
        4. Budgeting
        5. Evaluation — Peer Review
        6. Evaluation — Operations Audit
        7. Evaluation — Accounting Audit
    B. Operating Control Systems
        1. Patient Control
        2. Service Control
        3. Inventory Control
        4. Accounting
V. Information Processing Support Systems
    A. Communications
    B. Electronic Data Processing

Primary Medical Care Systems

All of the systems in an enterprise are oriented toward dispensing medical care. In a CHO, the objective is to keep people well, cure them, arrest disease if cure is impossible, and rehabilitate those who have suffered considerable physical damage. The key to all of this is primary medical care. To get medical services, a patient enters the system by visiting a primary care physician or other practitioner such as a dentist or psychiatrist. The primary care physician consults with the patient, examines him, makes a diagnosis, gives him treatment or refers him to a specialist, and follows up to see that he is treated. In doing this, the primary care physician employs supporting systems such as the services of a laboratory and the control systems of his business office.

The term primary care physician is coming into frequent use in HMO literature and requires some explanation in the context of systems operation. It refers to the role of generalist rather than specialist, or more broadly, to the person whom the patient goes to first for help with a problem. From a systems engineering point of view, the person the patient goes to first for help is the primary care practitioner. It follows then, that a specialist can perform the role of primary care physician as well as his own specialty as long as he is qualified for both. A primary care practitioner can be a general care dentist, a gynecologist handling pregnant women, a pediatrician handling children, or even a faith healer if used as the primary point of entry into a medical system. Thus, the term primary care provider is used to designate a system role rather than a professional class of practitioner.

Generally, a patient goes to a primary care practitioner by his own initiative. He waits until he needs medical care, or thinks he does, and initiates the action by making an appointment. For most people, it is the only way of getting into a care system. This is not true in CHOs. People in CHOs also receive care initiated by medical centers. In fact, preventive care is usually center initiated. This includes patient health education, inoculations, periodic physicals other preventive care. Health education is generally center initiated. Items of interest are distributed to patients by mail, and patients are often invited to courses of instruction. Patients are notified for inoculations and are called up when physicals are due. All of this is frequently controlled by a family health system in which a center provides health programs and sees that they are implemented.

Patient initiated care is rendered in office visits, home care, and outpatient visits. For office care, the patient makes an appointment with his own physician for a time when he can be scheduled. If his own physician is not available, an alternative is often suggested. When the patient is confined to his home, he may request home care — a doctor's visit or care administered by a visiting nurse. Finally, the patient can elect outpatient care.

One of the special features of CHOs, is the outpatient ward where patients can walk in for treatment without appointments. Outpatient care consists of treatment for minor accidents, mild infections, mild digestive disorders, and other disorders, including some kinds of minor surgery. The outpatient ward also includes emergency care when the patient may come in by himself or be brought in by ambulance.

Emergency care in some clinics is being expanded to full-fledged lifesaving systems.

Specialty Care Systems

Primary care providers refer patients for specialty care as needed—a situation that may arise out of patient initiated visits or center initiated annual physicals. The patient may be referred to a specialist physician, a therapist, a surgeon, or other provider. He may be booked into a hospital, an extended care facility, or a nursing home. Services are provided by the specialty providers with the knowledge of primary care providers. A health care center generally has a booking and follow-up system to assist primary care physicians in their referral work.

Patient Logistic Systems

One of the critical systems of a center is its patient handling system. Patients come to a center in several ways: by automobile, public transportation, foot, ambulance, and vehicles operated by a center. From the homes of patients to a center, within the center itself, and between the center and associated providers channels exist for handling patients. Facilities such as vehicles, parking space, and reception areas are established for the flow of patients. Centers are often located in convenient places and facilities are laid out to facilitate patient flow. Finally, the task of moving people efficiently is often controlled by a formal information system.

Medical Support and Other Systems

A number of systems providing medical support are sometimes available to primary care physicians. Some centers install and operate their own drug dispensing sytems—procure drugs in bulk form, mix them in accordance with prescription, and distribute them. Others enlist drug houses as associate providers. The same kind of arrangements are made for dispensing prosthetics such as eye glasses, hearing aids, etc. Most large centers operate special physical examination units, often run by parameds with a battery of devices arranged in stations to accumulate medical data on patients. Many centers have one or more laboratories to provide information about patients: chemical labs for running tests, x-ray labs for diagnosis, and backup laboratories either inhouse or under contract to handle special work such as multiphasic screening, unusual lab tests, and difficult radiology.

There are transportation systems to move patients, transport employees, and bring in medical supplies; supply systems that acquire, store, and distribute items of supply; facility systems for the acquisition, maintenance, and disposition of plant and equipment; and systems for hiring, training, deploying, and serving personnel.

Fiscal Systems

Each enterprise has a fiscal system which receives money, banks it, and makes payment to providers, employees and suppliers. In addition to regular transactions, a fiscal system includes the flow of funds for investment and a reverse flow as investments are repaid. Sources of funds include patients, benefactors paying for patients, and insurance companies. Payments are made in part or in whole through financial intermediaries who collect and remit funds to centers. Administrative systems, including billing, accounts payable and accounting help control the fiscal systems.

Operating and Technical Information Systems

Specialized medical information systems help providers. A center generally has a data system, which accumulates personal data and medical history on patients, arranges it, stores it, and retrieves it when needed. Some systems store medical procedures in a data bank for retrieval by diagnostically oriented selection procedures. Others do the same for drugs.

Very important are systems for accumulation, development and deployment of technical information, such as health technology, medical procedures, educational curricula, and training courses. Among centers, varying emphasis is placed on how much of this kind of intelligence is created inhouse or acquired outside. The systems include procedures for early distribution of vital data, and for storage of information in libraries or data banks.

Administrative Information Systems

Most centers have a full complement of administrative systems. There are two types: systems of management that translate broad objectives into operating results and systems that control operations at the operating level. The first set are vertical systems since they deal with flow of information up and down jurisdictional lines of organization. They include the formulation, promulgation, and feedback pertaining to policy, long-range planning, and short-range planning, the preparation of budgets, their dissemination, and reports on compliance. Finally, they include the periodic generation and distribution to management of information on how well a center operates, a peer review system in which medical care is compared against performance standards, a system to measure operating efficiency and utilization of capacity, and accounting audits to keep everyone honest.

Because quality is critical, the peer review systems are often thorough. In some centers, each practitioner is reviewed periodically by his fellows, and an independent agency is employed to see that it is done effectively. The outside agency conducts audits, certifies a center's practice, and referees disputes among peers over inspection findings.

The second set of administrative systems are horizontal: it deals with base level operations that cross jurisdictional lines. It includes systems that control processing of patients, services, inventories, money, and credit. Control systems for patients take many forms. Most providers operate their own booking systems for patient initiated services, augmented by a central system that takes over where individual systems leave off. The control systems often cover patients coming for center initiated services.

Service control systems operate in a similar way, each provider controlling his own services, with common services controlled by the center.

Some centers operate a family health system in which the health status of every enrollee is monitored through a computer recording patient history from which schedules for periodic examinations, inoculations, and follow-up treatment are determined.

Inventory control systems are generally operated by each practitioner of a center, augmented by a common system which controls the acquisition, storage, and distribution of common supplies and services.

Practitioners often keep their own accounting records, augmented to a greater or lesser degree by central systems that bill patients, pay suppliers, maintain journals and ledgers, and prepare operating reports.

Specialized Information Processing Systems

Finally, a center often provides practitioners with systems of communication and data processing. Systems of communication include telephone service with a central switchboard, paging systems and, in the more sophisticated centers, computer oriented telecommunication devices for booking patients, ordering supplies, and retrieving information from data banks. Electronic data processing systems perform patient booking, inventory control, billing and accounting, patient history taking, medical procedures selection, and drug selection.

A feature in the HMO blueprint is a linked data system. Such a system is built on modules of data that can form all information on transactions and status situations. The modules are conveyed by standardized codes that are machine readable and capable of generating families of compatible source documents, file records, and reports.

System Configuration. Systems come in many configurations. Large CHOs have many systems in complex configurations; small centers have fewer systems in simpler configurations. Surprisingly, configurations of small centers are often nearly as complex as those in large centers. The chief difference systemwise is not complexity, as one might suppose, but formality. In large centers, systems are frequently formalized and often automated, while in small ones they tend to be informal and hand-operated.

The configuration of systems in a care enterprise depends largely on the market it serves and the care it renders. Care in a center that serves a single community requires a system configuration different from one in a center serving many communities. Well-care systems differ considerably from sick-care systems.

When a large center is started from scratch, new systems have to be designed and installed. This is often the most difficult job in the development process, and the most costly. As a center grows, the point may be reached where inadequacy of systems arrests further growth. At this point, the center often redesigns its systems—a traumatic job that takes a long time.

There is little in the blueprint for CHOs that pertains to systems. However, the kind of care prescribed in the blueprint influences to a degree the kind of systems that must be established. Billing systems are partially determined by the billing requirements of third party payers, and certain record keeping systems are determined by PSRO requirements.

SUPPLY SOURCES

The basic systems of a health enterprise start with supply sources and end up with markets. A health care establishment in the broadest sense stretches from its supply sources to its markets — in a set of converging and diverging systems. While health care services are delivered from an establishment itself to multiple customers, resources flow to it in converging systems from multiple supply sources.

The most important source of supply for a care establishment is the neighborhood in which it is located, which usually supplies practitioners, employees, and most of the goods needed. For those goods that are not produced locally, suppliers can be found in the phone book. Most practitioners of a health care establishment come from the neighborhood. Often they are founders of a group or neighboring physicians who are induced to join after an establishment is created. There are many advantages of getting practitioners from the neighborhood: they are generally experienced, oriented, and bring their practices along with them. Other sources of practitioners are universities, hospitals, and practices of practitioners seeking new connections — most of which are out-of-town.

Employees are generally available in the neighborhood. The exceptions, unfortunately, are the higher skilled employees. Nurses, parameds, and administrators are often not available locally and must be sought elsewhere.

Almost everything else can be purchased locally or attained through national or regional suppliers, with the exception of money, which unlocks the other sources. The best source of money is surplus earnings or profits on operations. Often, earnings are insufficient for development needs and other sources must be sought. Alternative sources of investment capital are the principals, the local bank, an investment house, private placement groups, public issue and government.

The supply sources structure of an enterprise depends largely on its make-or-buy policy. Some resources must reside inhouse, others out-of-house, while some are optional in that they can reside inhouse or remain outside. Resources used inside an establishment are its employees, equipment, and principals. Resources that mainly reside outside are power generating equipment, intercity transportation equipment, and equipment of major service suppliers. A health care enterprise gets the benefit of an outside resource by purchasing the services it produces — as it does when it buys electric power and telephone services. A breakdown of resources according to whether they must reside inhouse, outside, or in either place is shown in Table 5-2.

TABLE 5-2
Location of Various Resource Capabilities

Resource Output	Inside	Outside	Optional
Primary care	x		
Specialty care			x
Lab services			x
Pharmacy			x
Multiphasic testing			x
Building operation	x		
External transportation			x
Internal transportation	x		
Supply	x		
Maintenance			x
Electric power and heat		x	
Telephone		x	
Intercom			x
Risk taking			x
Financing			x
Data processing			x
Administrative services			
Basic	x		
Other			x
Space	x		

The source options are many. Indeed, it is interesting to note they outnumber mandatory items, and that the number of resources that must be located within an enterprise are relatively few. Furthermore, there are optional ways of acquiring inside resources. Practitioners and others can be engaged as principals or can be employed. Routine workers, however, are generally employed, or hired from outside agencies. In some cases, entire management teams are hired.

All of the inside facilities can be purchased or leased. With everything leased, the investment costs of a center are kept to a minimum. Special deals of a joint venturing nature are often made to

attain resources either internally or externally. Some arrangements
are as follows:

- Hospitals and other medical suppliers coventure
  with health care establishments.
- Insurance companies underwrite all or part of
  risks involved in operation.
- Service corporations coventure or provide services
  for a fee or for a share of revenues.
- Investment groups provide all or part of the
  capital for fees or part of the action.

The blueprint for CHOs is relatively flexible on resources. HMO provisions call for an inhouse primary care capability and ability to administer a prepaid plan. They also require the plan organization to be
nonprofit, though the restriction is not extended to coventuring units.
Finally, they restrict the amount of risk that can be assumed by outside insurance companies.

Thus, the anatomical model of group practice is complex. It covers a
range of practices from three-man groups to supercomplexes like
Kaiser. Complexity arises out of combinations that can be created,
given the number of optional features available. These features can
make a significant difference in the effectiveness of a center. Those
centers fortunate enough to make the right development decisions are
efficient and prosperous; the others have growing pains. It is,
therefore, important to consider the options with a knowledge of alternative structure.

Chapter 6

Alternative Structuring

Alternative structuring distinguishes one establishment from another. Some are centralized, while others are decentralized; some are rigid in approach, while others are flexible; some are comprehensive, while others are specialized; some are concentrated, while others are spread out. Though most have common elements, there is a difference in the way they are put together. Some structuring must be fashioned in certain ways to attain the diverse objectives of health care enterprises. Other structuring is optional, dependent upon the whims of principals and chance factors.

Optional structuring determines the welfare of an establishment, i.e., the selection of correct alternatives is pivotal. What are the critical alternatives and what are the criteria for selecting them?

Not all alternative decisions are critical. Many make little difference. There are often several answers that are acceptable. However, if consistently wrong decisions are made, the consequences can be devastating. Critical alternatives involve the structuring of:

- Service Line
- Organization
- Fiscal and Financial Systems

Criteria for selection among alternatives are grounded in three sets of information: (1) the HMO formula, (2) the CHO blueprint, and (3) general economic theory tempered by humanistic considerations. HMO legislation provides a legalistic blueprint that contains options. It also has restrictions that many consider economically unsound. In spite of the restrictions, there are some advantages in staying within the HMO blueprint: favored treatment by the government; good positioning in the event of nationalization of the health care industry; better public relations, including a favorable press; and better union relations. But, there are also disadvantages which include a formula that is not always workable and the fact that many practitioners would not, under any circumstances, join an HMO.

Somewhat broader than the HMO formula is the blueprint for comprehensive care establishments that has evolved out of customary practices. It should be noted that few CHOs are qualified HMOs. In fact, the term CHO is used to distinguish this type of organization from the HMO, which is just one kind of CHO. The broader CHO blueprint is needed if large numbers of health care centers are to be created. It is likely that Congress will eventually adopt this blueprint for HMOs. When it does, HMOs and CHOs will be one and the same; and the choice of one name or the other will make little difference. At the present time, however, there is a significant difference between the two.

Not that the CHO blueprint is vastly broader than the HMO prescription; it is not. CHOs have the same specific objectives as HMOs and adopt many of the same practices specified in legislation. Where the blueprints differ is on practical features. For example, the CHO formula does *not* :

- Prescribe a definite care package.
- Try to make employees out of physicians.
- Insist on open enrollment.
- Require capitation payment.
- Require capitation risk on the part of principals.
- Require nonprofit status.
- Require consumer representation on boards of directors.

In most other respects, the CHO formula is like that of the HMO. It permits, though it doesn't require, all of the HMO prescriptions; and a non-HMO formulated in accordance with the CHO blueprint can be readily converted to a HMO if legislation should later mandate it.

Thus, there are advantages in adopting the CHO blueprint as a guideline. It is likely to provide economic advantages not attainable under the HMO blueprint, and it specifies configurations that can be easily converted to an HMO. The disadvantage is that even the broader blueprint can be too restrictive. Most group practices today couldn't live with it except as a long range objective.

The third level of criteria goes beyond the broader CHO blueprint. It constrains choice only by economic considerations tempered by human factors. In the final analysis, a practice need only be economical and acceptable to its principals.

Thus, one must consider three levels of criteria which require some priority structuring. Logic dictates that the priority structuring go from the broadest to the narrowest criteria. Above all, a practice must be economical enough to sustain itself and grow. Within this broad criteria, the CHO blueprint can be applied, and within CHO limitations, consideration might be given to aspects of the narrower HMO blueprint.

SERVICE LINE ALTERNATIVES

Decisions on the line of health care services delivered to patients determine the basic character of a center. Decisions on its lines of support services determine the success of the center.

Health Care Services

The most influential decision that a group makes is usually made for them — whether to go single specialty or multispecialty. If the physicians joining a group happen to be in the same specialty, chances are they will go single specialty without giving the matter a second thought. And if they are a widely respected group, their decision — or lack of it — probably is correct. There are distinct advantages as well as disadvantages of single specialty practice. Both are listed below:

Advantages and Disadvantages of Single Specialty Practice

Advantages

- Concentration of talent
- High learning potential
- Good consultation capability
- Mutual understanding of problems
- High interchangeability among practitioners.

Disadvantages

- Reliance on referrals
- Thin market
- Patient inconvenience
- Danger of losing market to CHOs.

For a competent group with a widespread reputation, the advantages loom large, the disadvantages, small. When the situation reverses, it is time to reconsider.

In contrast with decisions on going single specialty, a decision to provide multispecialty care often requires a lot of thought. Practitioners of different specialties do not naturally congregate as those in the same specialty do. They consider how their practices will merge and explore the market for their collective specialties. At the least, they attempt to balance the provider team to match the spectrum of patient needs.

The distinct advantages and disadvantages of multispecialty practice are listed below:

Advantages and Disadvantages of Multispecialty Practice

Advantages

- Interpractice consultation opportunities
- Wide spectrum of care available
- Patient convenience
- More concentrated market.

Disadvantages

- Limited specialty capability
- Limited practitioner cohesiveness
- Limited interchangeability of practitioners
- Limited intrapractice consultation.

Multispecialty groups make more decisions about service line than their single specialty cognates. A set of thorny decisions arises concerning extent of care given. At one extreme, a group can give sick care, with each specialist sticking to his own business. At the other extreme, a group can provide just about everything from medicine to rat control guidance. In between the two extremes, there is a continuous and dense distribution of care packages. An example of the range is presented in Table 6-1.

As multispecialty groups grow both in size and comprehensiveness of service, they face more decisions on how to structure operations.

TABLE 6-1
Limited vs. Extended Care

Package Item	Limited Package	Extended Package
Sick care	Yes	Yes
Well care	No	Yes
Regular checkups	No	Yes
Inoculation programs	No	Yes
Patient education programs	No	Yes
Primary care	Yes	Yes
Surgical care	No	Yes
Inpatient care — short term	No	Yes
Inpatient care — extended	No	Yes
Psychological care	No	Yes
Special therapy	No	Yes
Dental care	No	Yes
Optometry	No	Yes
Pharmacy	No	Yes
Regular office care	Yes	Yes
Outpatient care	No	Yes
Emergency care	No	Yes
Home care (regular)	No	Yes

Two alternatives encountered are:

- Should initiation of routine care such as periodic examinations be left to the patient or the center?
- Should conventional patient processing systems be retained or a more streamlined one adopted?

Selection of alternative packages and methods of delivery obviously raise thorny problems. Each health care establishment has to work out these problems as they arise. They should recognize when the time comes to make changes, know the alternatives, and carefully consider the various consequences.

The following ground rules are useful:

1. Single speciality groups that have trouble keeping up revenues should consider converting to multispecialty practice.

2. Multispecialty groups that have trouble keeping up revenues should consider enlarging their care packages.

3. Limited care groups should consider enlarging care packages in order to give better health care to patients and to preclude invasion of the local market by competitors.

4. Groups that adopt comprehensive care should consider streamlining patient processing.

The streamlining of patient processing runs into cherished principles long honored in medical practice. Most cherished of all is maintaining the patient-physician relationship. Not only do physicians cherish this relationship, but patients do also. Streamlining the flow of patients in a clinic is severely limited when physician-patient relationships are maintained. The alternatives are to do away with the relationship or build around it. Most clinics choose to build around it—a wise approach—since patient processing can be considerably streamlined without severely altering the relationships.

Another cherished principle is to avoid mass processing of patients. In the parlance of systems engineers, medicine is largely a job shop operation, not an assembly line one. Sick care lends itself to the job shop approach. The patient initiates a visit by calling for an appointment, comes in at the appointed time, and sees his doctor after waiting for others with prior appointments. He is taken into the treatment area, given essential care by the doctor, and dismissed—much like a car in a repair shop that is processed in one stage on an individual basis.

Well-care, on the other hand, lends itself to more streamlined processing. Patients are scheduled for their annuals by a clinic. They come in, get in line, and go through a battery of test procedures—similar to an assembly line basis. Patient education is also scheduled and conducted in groups. In fact, most well-care is handled by semi-mass-processing methods of this kind.

As clinics grow they tend to specialize. The outpatient ward within clinics was created to streamline care. Minor accidents and upsets are treated in outpatient wards—convenient for patients and a relief to overloaded physician offices. Emergency care and home health care systems are being devised by growing clinics.

Finally, with many ways of entering the system, each followed by a distinct processing system, the modern clinic has special control systems for booking and scheduling both patients and treatment. The triage procedure is one approach. Patients who come into a center on their own initiative, or the center's, are sorted out and put into the right channels — generally with an effort to maintain the physician-patient relationship.

Various ways of processing patients arise in the life-course of a practice. Good general guidelines for decisionmaking in this area are to adopt all procedures that make care more economical or convenient for patients while maintaining the physician-patient relationship and keeping a high quality of care.

Support Services

Alternative support services present another series of decisions. At different points in the life of a clinic, it should consider whether to set up inhouse capability for support services that it buys outside. Not only is it sometimes cheaper to buy, but inhouse support services are handy and controllable. Support services that often require such considerations are:

- Clinic Lab Service
- Diagnostic X-Ray
- Multiphasic Screening
- Dental Lab Service

The size of the clinic is the major criterion for providing these services inhouse. Table 6-2 presents a rough guide for the decisions involved.

TABLE 6-2
Clinic Size Criterion for Inhouse
Medical Support Services

Medical Support Services	Personnel Required Per 1,000 Patients		Minimum Force	
	Office Practice Only	Office & Hospital	Partial Service	Full Service
Clinical lab	0.5	1.5	1.0	30.0
Diagnostic x-ray	0.4	1.2	1.0	5.0
Multiphasic screening	0.2	1.6	- 1.0 to	30.0
Dental lab	0.1	0.3	1.0	5.0

Groups have stat labs for quick and dirty tests like cultures, urine analysis and blood counts. In fact, as the table shows, 1.5 thousand patients are all that are necessary to justify a lab technician, and only 1.0 technician is necessary to man a limited service lab. Many thousands of patients are needed, however, to fully utilize a full-scale clinical laboratory. According to Table 6-2, it takes a 20,000-patient clinic with hospital services or three 20,000-patient office-practice-only clinics to keep a full-fledged laboratory busy.

An office practice can afford an x-ray technician after it has several thousand patients, and a full-fledged diagnostic x-ray group when it has more than 12.5 thousand patients. Ten thousand dental patients can keep a dental lab technician busy; 50,000 are needed for a full service dental laboratory.

Multiphasic screening units require from 5,000 to 150,000 patients, depending upon the automation employed. A complete multiphasic unit can be operated by one person with an investment in equipment of $15,000. Large automated centers, with investment ranging from $500,000 to $1.0 million, require fifteen or more people for operation and large numbers of patients to keep them busy. A large-sized multiphasic unit can serve ten 20,000-patient, office-practice-only clinics.

As clinics get bigger, alternatives for processing information arise. At various points, consideration should be given to computerization of the following systems:

- Diagnostic analysis
- Procedure lookup
- Drug lookup
- Patient history records

Several companies merchandize computerized procedures for analyzing multiphasic test results on a variety of body screens. The computer reads test results, adjusts it for special conditions and characteristics of the patient, and makes a diagnosis from the adjusted data. Medi-Comp of Cleveland has been doing this for years at a cost of about $2.00 per analysis. Other computers read x-rays, cardiograms, encephalograms, and other electronically recorded data. They look up medical procedures and drugs and keep patient history records. The new procedures improve practice by extending the intellectual reach of practitioners.

Opportunities are emerging for improving mundane procedures such as booking, billing, and bookkeeping. In their growth, clinics reach the point at which billing and bookkeeping can best be done in specialized service units. The scheduling of well-care can also be done more economically in scheduling units.

Booking patients for conventional care is often left to individual physicians since they generally do it better than others. Some clinics use timeshared computers that allow physicians to do their own booking at remote terminals, thus providing both the economies of central service and booking automony in one system.

In addition to alternative information systems, clinics must consider alternative levels of mechanization. There is always a question about how much to automate. Every system has a range of configurations; and some systems have configurations ranging from pen-and-ink procedures to full automation. At the automation end of the spectrum, there are at least three basic kinds of mechanized processing: (1) service bureau processing, (2) timesharing network, and (3) inhouse computer.

Alternatives for developing information systems are so complex, it is almost impossible to prepare a general strategy regarding them. A few guidelines, however, are available:

- The systems of small health care centers — 10,000 or fewer enrollees — should be kept relatively informal, decentralized, and lightly mechanized, using service bureau and outside timesharing for computer backup.
- Large clinics — 50,000 or more enrollees — should have systems that are relatively formalized, centralized, and mechanized by outside timesharing and inhouse computers. Table 6-3 shows these systems characteristics and how they should range from small to large clinics — with systems characteristics of intermediate-sized clinics interpolated between the extremes.
- Formalization, automation and centralization of information systems are developments that have no virtue other than the economies they afford. They are expensive and create systems that are inflexible. In fact, side effects of systematizing are often so destructive, it behooves decision makers to place a heavy burden of proof on demonstrating economies.
- In the centralization process, there is a tendency to take away decisionmaking from practitioners where it generally belongs and place it with administrative people. This can be avoided by remote control systems that have centralized routine functions along with decentralized decisionmaking.
- In the treacherous areas of developing systems, it pays to employ

TABLE 6-3
Desired Information
Systems Characteristics

Systems Characteristics	Small Center	Large Center
Formalization	Little	Much
Automation	Little	Much
Centralization	Little	Much
Service bureau	Frequently	Sometimes
Timesharing network	Sometimes	Somtimes
Inhouse computer	Seldom	Frequently

management consultants for professional advice before making critical decisions.

ORGANIZATION ALTERNATIVES

There are significant organization alternatives. Some deal with legal forms, others with basic structure.

Basic Organization Options

Health care groups are organized in one of two basic ways: (1) as an integrated organization—a single corporation, partnership, or individual enterprise: (2) as a federated association of independent providers joined under contract to form a cohesive operation. In the integrated organization, practitioners usually work for salary. They come to work at specified hours, do their jobs, and go home at the end of the day. Like other employees, they receive fringe benefits such as paid vacations, life and health insurance, income sharing, and retirement income.

In contrast, the professionals of a federated organization maintain their independent status. They generally charge fees for each service, and sometimes share capitation gains and losses. Usually they work under medical plans instead of employment contracts. They devote a stipulated amount of time to enrollees and abide by policies, rules and regulations of the group. Otherwise, they are free to come and go as they please, treat nonenrollees as well as enrollees, and in almost every other way, enjoy the privileges of professional independence.

Both kinds of basic organization have their advantages. The integrated organization can be aligned with greater precision, given stronger lines of authority, and tighter controls. It is despotic to a degree. Given strong and wise leadership and employees who are willing to conform, it could do better than the looser federation. A federation, on the other hand, is more likely to succeed than an integrated group, especially if it has self-starting, self-disciplined providers. Furthermore, the federated group is easier to organize because it is more attractive to physicians.

Executive functions in each kind of organization are usually performed by a board of trustees and an executive staff. The board creates the establishment, sets its objectives, obtains critical intelligence about it, approves development plans and capital budgets, acquires investment funds, and sees that objectives are met. The executive staff implements objectives of trustees. It creates relationships with providers and the public, administers capital budgets, acquires resources, and sees that the establishment operates properly.

Committees help boards in the following ways: executive committees act for boards when they are adjourned; medical committees establish clinical standards; public service committees represent patients and others in policy making; financial committees obtain and budget funds; and review committees audit centers for conformance with policy.

There is a difference between the executive structures of integrated organization, and those of federations. In the integrated establishment, executive structure is formal; in federations, it is informal and sometimes almost invisible. A comparison of the types is shown in Table 6-4.

Foundations for medical care make up a special kind of federated group, one that has evolved out of solo practice to give patients comprehensive care. They have centralized plan organizations, but their medical centers are dispersed. In fact, the medical centers are simply the office suites of former solo practitioners.

TABLE 6-4
Executive Structure Integrated
vs. Federated Establishments

Item	Integrated	Federated
Policy	Formal	Informal
Committees	Many	Few
Control Structure	Centralized	Decentralized
Executive Office	Large	Small
Planning	Centralized	Decentralized
Regulations	Many	Few
Discipline	Centralized	Self-Imposed

Foundations are organized to accommodate their peculiar physical layouts. Since the medical units are dispersed, organization is decentralized. Because of their distinctive configurations, foundations have the following advantages and disadvantages:

Advantages

1. They are easy to create since they combine practitioners already in place.
2. Good use is made of pre-existing practices.
3. Wide area coverage is achieved.
4. They provide the most entry points per practitioner, saving travel time both of patients and doctors.
5. They are flexible.
6. A high degree of practitioner freedom is achieved.
7. They are acceptable to many practitioners who reject other kinds of CHOs.

Disadvantages

1. Patients get shuffled around more than in integrated centers.
2. There is less peer contact for practioners.
3. Special talent is spread thin.
4. Support services are spread thin.
5. Equipment is spread thin.
6. There is less control over quality of care.

The way that functions of an organization are combined into operating sections, groups, and departments depends on several factors: size of the group, mix of services, do/buy arrangements,* geographical distribution, personalities, status, and established prerogatives. Organization experts have ground rules for combining functions, and these should be heeded if a center is to be successful. But, more often than not, they are honored in the breach.

Functions are, or should be, combined in jurisdictional groups along organization lines — lines of authority and communications that link trustees with operating levels. Functions that are alike are often combined to form *colony type organization*. Functions not necessarily alike but integrated systemwise are sometimes combined to form a *line organization*. Both kinds of organization are used, but colony groupings predominate.

Much of the medical industry is in an early stage of industrialization where one, two, or three-person organizations perform a variety of tasks with little specialization. The small establishments are, of necessity, colony style, and they have come to accept this style as the only way to organize. Straight line organization, often called assembly line medicine, is shunned by many physicians and, therefore, will take time for wide acceptance. Moreover, line organization is suited only to certain phases of preventive care and requires a large volume of patients for economic operation.

Physical layout has a lot to do with how functions are grouped. A centralized center is organized differently than one that is decentralized, a center with satellites differently than one without, a two-facility center differently than one with a single facility, etc.

Regardless of the basic type of organization, operating functions should be grouped along relatively clearcut organizational lines where each individual has one person to whom he is responsible and from whom he gets necessary resources. Organized in this way, a center has unbroken lines of authority and responsibility from board to operating level, a two-way channel of communications up and down these lines, and two-way channels of exchange in which funds are budgeted and results obtained. In an integrated group, organizational lines are quite obvious, sometimes long, and configured in a steep hierarchy. While in a federation, the lines are subtle, if not subliminal, the configuration — if hierarchical at all — is flat, and lines of authority and responsibility are limited in functional scope, frequently punctuated by units operating with much autonomy.

---

*Do/buy arrangements refer to what is done inhouse versus what is bought outside.

In evolvement of organization structure, junction points occur where decision makers have to take one course or another. The most difficult choices deal with how to delegate duties of professionals to paraprofessionals. The subject of delegation is being debated in the public forum. The basic issue has two diametrical points of view. Many professionals frown on delegation of customary physician duties; others think it is a great idea.

Qualified paraprofessionals can relieve physicians and other professionals of duties. The law allows it, and it is done successfully both in private practices and in the armed forces. Moreover, the practice has been accepted by the federal government, promoted by it, and is spreading, as parameds are trained in government-sponsored educational programs. Parameds have been trained to take over most of the duties of physicians. In routine duties, they often do better than physicians because of repetition and because they don't get bored with routine work as easily as physicians do. Patients apparently accept them and some patients even prefer them for routine care.

The advantage of the paramed is that he or she frees the doctor to spend more time on critical care. Further, a doctor with a paramed can see nearly twice as many patients in a day as he can without one. Work is divided between the two so that the doctor handles the critical care while the paramed handles the routine. Physicians even supervise the work of three or four parameds; but in such situations, the parameds too often get into critical care. It is when parameds get into critical care that serious questions arise about delegation. In fact, the whole issue can be boiled down to a critical ratio— *the number of parameds per doctor.* Should the number be 0, 1:4, 1:2, 1, 2, 4 or 8? At one end of the scale, no parameds are used; at the other end, physicians do little but supervise parameds.

Delegation to parameds can be pivotal. On the one hand, it extends available physicians, reduces costs of care, and in proper proportion, improves care. On the other hand, it is difficult to control, adds risk, makes an establishment more vulnerable to lawsuit, and, if carried too far, destroys the professionalism of a medical practice. As parameds per physician increases, the critical duties of parameds also increase. At some point in the progression, parameds go beyond their depth and require almost constant supervision. At that point, they become "troops" rather than underprofessionals. The doctors, in turn, become supervisors rather than professional doers. Furthermore, as supervisors, they lose their touch, both figuratively and literally. And professionalism disappears.

Precursor analysis of this is found in the legal and auditing professions which have been delegating professional duties for a decade. It is getting to the point where few lawyers can try a case, and few auditors can check a set of books. Excessive delegation does eventually destroy professionalism.

Finally, there are many kinds of organization styles. There are top-dominated organizations, which have one-sided relationships biased toward the top, orders of prestige graduated upward from bottom to top, and systems of compensation to match the hierarchy. In contrast, there are professional style organizations with balanced relationships between components, where place in the organization hierarchy has no special prestige, no effect on bargaining power or compensation. Often a professional style organization has a reverse order of status where many of those at the operating level have more prestige, bargaining power, and compensation than those at the top. Examples involve the professional athlete, movie star, research scientist, and some medical practitioners.

In between, there are hybrids of extremes. Because the medical industry is largely composed of professional doers, professional style organization is widespread. Since many organizational alternatives must be considered as a practice grows, the question which arises is: How does the health care executive decide which course to take?

At many decision junctions, the course is determined by circumstances, since structure and style are largely controlled by underlying systems of care. However, there is some leeway in the selection process. The following ground rules for basic organization provide rough criteria for selecting among alternative forms:

- Organize to accommodate systems of care.
- Keep decisionmaking as decentralized as possible.
- Put the burden of economic proof on proposals to centralize operations.
- Use parameds up to but not including the point where they need significant supervision.
- Adopt the style of organization that best suits the key personnel involved.

Legal Forms of Organization

Legal forms of organization are available for any kind of basic organization. What is more, there are often several kinds that can be adopted for a given situation. On occasion, it may be desirable to change the basic structure of an organization to accommodate a legal form, but generally the situation is reversed: one mainly selects legal forms to fit operating structures.

A single enterprise can have several legal forms of organization. For example, a holding company, or other association, can have many subsidiaries, each with a legal form different from the others. Federations of providers sometimes involve enough legal forms to astound a corporation lawyer. There are forms for income producing entitities: proprietorships, partnerships, and corporations; and forms for managing property: estate trusts, conventional investment trusts, and REITs. Each family of legal forms comes in a variety which keeps at least two kinds of lawyers busy full time.

The income producing forms of organization are described in textbooks on business practice and corporate finance. Some of these books are well organized and in a few hundred pages cover about 90% of the field. Unfortunately, the 10% not covered is often germane in a specific situation, and it takes volumes, that only lawyers can afford to master, to expound on the last 10%.

The legal forms of organization are employed to classify enterprises for public regulation; proprietorships get one kind of treatment, corporations, another, etc. In addition, each legal form has one or more specific purposes, such as prescribing how principles of an enterprise relate to one another, how continuity of an enterprise can be maintained, and how its assets can be transferred between principals. Some legal forms call for centralized management, limitation of liability, profit making, dividend payments, and employee benefits. All of them deal with taxation — which has the most influence on choice of organization.

Table 6-5 relates ten important organization features with major types of legal enterprise.

While all enterprises have a legal form by which they are classified for taxation and regulation, not all are chartered by legal documents. Proprietorships more often than not operate without formal documentation other than registration numbers filed with the IRS or other branches of government. Partnerships are often created with a handshake, and some associations that behave like corporations do not have charters at all. However, most corporations do have charters, just as partnerships have partnership agreements, and proprietorships maintain some identification documentation.

Trust arrangements are proliferating in the medical industry. They are not only a convenient way to manage property, but they are often used to cut down taxes. Estate building today is almost entirely done by means of trusts because of tax exemptions. A typical health care establishment is likely to have an assortment of group and individual

TABLE 6-5
**Organization Features by
Legal Types of Enterprise**

Features			Legal Types of Enterprise			
	Proprie-torship	Partner-ship	Corporation			
			Basic for Profit	Tax Option	Prof. Svc.	Non-Profit
Associates	No	Yes	Yes	Yes	Yes	Yes
Centralized management	No	Limited	Yes	Limited	Limited	Yes
Legal continuity	No	No	Yes	Yes	Yes	Yes
Transfer of assets	No	No	Yes	Yes	Yes	Yes
Limited liability	No	No[1]	Yes	Yes	No	Yes
Profit making potential	Yes	No	Yes	Yes	Yes	No
Corporate income tax	No	No[1]	Yes	No	Yes	No
Tax exemptions	Few	Few	Many	Many	Many	Many
Benefits potential	Small	Small	Large	Large	Large	Large
Regulation	Little	Little	Much	Much	Much	Much

[1] Limited partnerships are an exception.

trusts for handling profit sharing, retirement programs, insurance, and other programs. Physicians in high brackets take advantage of investment and family trusts to build up estates; and selection of alternatives often determines their degree of success.

Nonprofit Organizations

Nonprofit corporations are not what they seem to be to people unfamiliar with them. They are widely regarded, especially by government people, as sacrosanct, presumably because they have lofty ideals in place of profit motives. Actually, they are somewhat of a ripoff. To survive and grow, they must make a "profit" or be forever supported by patrons. Most of them do make a "profit," but it is concealed in the jargon of institutional accounting. The major difference between the nonprofit and for-profit organizations is that nonprofits don't pay income tax. The for-profit corporations do have an advantage, otherwise there wouldn't be many of them. They can issue stock and pay dividends. In this way, their stockholders can profit both from earnings and from speculative gains when stock is traded. Investors like stocks, and in spite of corporate income taxes, invest heavily in them. The profit making corporations rely on stock purchases for much of their growth capital.

Nonprofits, on the other hand, often scrounge around for investment capital. They rely on grants and charitable contributions. They also raise investment capital by loans and by generating operating surpluses.

Government provides advantages for the nonprofits. In addition to grants, it gives them service contracts, guarantees their loans, and extends favored tax treatment such as tax exemption for their bondholders. Almost half of the hospital bonds issued in 1975 were exempt from federal tax. The exemptions cut about 25% off the interest they pay. Exemptions come about by financing medical facilities through state and municipal authorities. For these reasons, many health care establishments are set up as nonprofit corporations. They can raise capital without issuing stock while enjoying the advantages of nonprofit status.

Those that go nonprofit have two main choices: They can become 501-C-3 corporations or 501-C-4s. The C-3 franchises are more difficult to get, but they are preferred because C-3 corporations can bestow tax exempt status on grants and donations given to them, while the C-4s cannot.

Under the blueprint for HMOs, the plan organization must be a nonprofit association. Although this is not specified in the act, in practice it works out that way—at least in most states. Furthermore, the plan organization must have consumer representation on the board of trustees.

To have or not to have consumer representation on the board of a health care establishment is an alternative that usually has to be faced at some time. Consumer representatives often are troublemakers. However, good consumer representatives contribute much to a board. One problem with the whole concept of consumer representation is to find people who really represent the consumer. Labor leaders and civil rights leaders often vie for that distinction. Determining what consumers want as a group is an art in itself, and it is not at all certain that "public figures" can do that.

Profit Organizations

In a federated group, each unit can have its own legal form. There are nonprofit plan organizations that bind together almost every kind of legal entity — physicians set up as proprietors, partners, and professional corporations; service units as profit corporations, etc. Most combinations have apparently been explored. The best of both worlds is frequently attained by judicious combination of nonprofit and profit forms.

A popular form used by groups of physicians is the tax option corporation. It has most of the advantages of a corporation, while at the same time, it allows principals to be taxed as partners to avoid the corporation tax. Tax option companies are restricted to ten stockholders. While profits are passed through without corporate taxation, profit sharing and retirement plans in tax option groups are severely limited.

Except for tax option corporations, the profit sharing and retirement plans of corporations are more liberal than in partnerships and proprietorships. For all intents and purposes, noncorporate entities are restricted to Keogh-type plans which limit the tax exempt amounts that a person can put away yearly to 15% of salary or $7,500, whichever is the lower. The upper limit of corporate plans is $75,000 and 100% of earnings subject to a complex set of rules for qualifying that keeps tax exemptions well within the maximum limits but not as low as Keogh.

In recent years, many practitioners set up professional corporations, or PCs, a relatively new legal form adopted by all states. It allows qualified professionals of all disciplines to create corporations in which the professionals serve as principals, whereas previously they could not incorporate in most states. The PC has restrictions. Stock can be owned only by the practicing professionals, and the usual corporate limits on liability are waived. In return for these trade-offs, PCs get the liberal retirement plan opportunities of corporations.

Cooperatives are used successfully for health care organizations. One of the largest and most successful cooperatives is Group Health Cooperative of Puget Sound, which has several hundred thousand enrollees. Cooperatives have the advantage of getting "true" consumer representation and a source of investment funding not usually tapped by other kinds of organizations.

Employee owned corporations are beginning to appear in the medical industry. Actually PCs are a form of employee owned establishments; but there are others as well for payroll employees. In a federated setup, the service unit of a CHO can be employee owned.

The employee owned corporation opens up employees as a source of capital. It also introduces unusual incentives for efficiency — desirable in parts of the medical industry dominated by strong unions. Some planners are looking into this kind of organization to rescue failing hospitals.

Criteria for Selection of Legal Forms

The right combination of legal formations can significantly influence a health care enterprise. It can affect morale, incentives to produce, taxes paid, estate building capability, vulnerability to suits and regulation, and ability to raise capital. As situations change, opportunities are frequently available for changes in the legal structure of an organization.

Consider, for example, an integrated CHO that operates as a nonprofit corporation. It has trouble attracting good physicians because employment is all it has to offer them. Because of union activity, its hospital costs are out of line. Just before going under, it switches to a federated organization. The health plan unit remains a nonprofit organization. Facilities are spun off to a profit making corporation that leases them back. The hospital employees organize an employee owned organization. Physicians form their own organizational units, some as individual enterprises, others as partners, and the remainder in a PC.

Under the new setup, everybody gains something. The employees of the hospital cut out featherbedding and save enough to cut down costs and raise salaries. The physicians get more professional freedom and pay less income taxes. The service corporation that takes over the facilities makes out well. And so it goes. A new combination of arrangements involving both basic organization structure and legal forms makes the difference between success and failure.

An enterprise in an entirely different setting might do the same thing in reverse, going from a loose federation to an integrated group, with similar but opposite changes in legal structure, and with equal success. Others making less dramatic changes might also enjoy equal success.

The potential for improving operations through legal forms is great. The question is how to do it. Alternatives for changing legal forms are almost always present, and opportunities to do so can arise at any time. So the most important thing to do is to keep vigilant for the opportunities and recognize them when they arise. This is an art in itself, and often requires the support of qualified professionals, as does the job of making changes.

Professional help can be obtained from a good tax man who knows law, or a good lawyer who knows taxes. Lucky is the enterprise that has both. Periodically, and at times when changes are made in basic conditions, organization forms should be reviewed by professionals.

The rough criteria for choosing legal organizational forms are:

1. Satisfy the mandatory factors such as:
   A. Conformance with law
   B. Requirements of principals
   C. Preferences of investors
2. Choose legal structure to accommodate basic structure rather than the other way around — except where trade-offs are large enough to clearly justify the reverse approach.
3. Keep in mind objectives which are to:
   A. Inspire morale
   B. Minimize taxes
   C. Minimize liability
   D. Improve benefits programs
   E. Improve public acceptance.
4. Be sure that the legal structures are formalized and documented.
5. Get professional consultation and assistance.

FISCAL AND FINANCIAL SYSTEMS ALTERNATIVES

Alternatives exist for handling fiscal and financial affairs of a health care enterprise. The choice is often critical. There are alternatives for charging patients, paying practitioners, controlling expenses, and handling funds — all pertaining to revenues and expenses. There are risk taking alternatives, different packages of fringe benefits, and diverse ways to finance startup and subsequent development.

Revenue and Expense System Alternatives

For a long time physicians got paid a fee for each service — mainly in cash. This was a convenient form of payment for a few reasons: no bad checks and simple bookkeeping. Although the system still exists, it is declining and may soon become extinct. Instead of cash, people pay by check. Rather than pay on the spot, they prefer to be billed for later payment; often third party payment replaces self-pay. The modern practice center, which is involved with all these forms of payment, has a choice.

The methods of payment are closely related to markets and classes of patients. People who walk into a clinic for sick care often pay cash for each service rendered, on the spot, or after being billed. Some have insurance policies that pay part of the bill. The health care establishment has the choice of processing the insurance claims for the patient, or letting him do it himself. More practices are taking on this chore for patients since they have to fill out the medical portions of claims anyway. In fact, the trend is so strong, the cost of clerical work is going up as practices hire people just to fill out insurance forms.

Methods of payment are related to programs of care. Benefactors prescribe charging and collection methods, and each package of care required has a tailor made method of payment along with it. So an assortment of payment alternatives exists that relates to health care packages. Since each benefactor and third party payer has his own pet package, a large health care establishment finds itself with a half dozen different kinds of payment plans to service.

Alternative Prepayment Plans

The big benefactors, such as Medicare and Medicaid, generally make up their own packages; practitioners can take them or leave them, if they qualify. However, CHOs also develop their own plans. There is a continuous range of payment plan possibilities providing many future alternatives. Although payment plans have a common structure, several variations (as shown in Table 6-6) account for the many possibilities:

TABLE 6-6
Prepayment Plan Variations

SCOPE:	Office care, Inpatient care, etc.
FAMILY RATES:	By the person, family of 3, 4, 5, etc.
DEDUCTIBLES:	Across-the-board, limited, none. 0%, 10%, 20%, . . .
COPAYMENTS:	Across-the-board, limited, none. 0%, 10%, 20%, . . .
ADD-ONS:	Office visits, house calls, etc.
SPECIAL RATES:	Elderly, Medicaid, Medicare, etc.

Payment plans are often tailored to yield a competitive rate. With the cost of medical care running $500 per person, a family of three would pay $1,500 annually, much more than most families, or their employers, are willing to pay. The cost is usually trimmed from 30% to 50% by limiting the basic care package itself, and by using copayments, deductible, and add-ons. A comprehensive care package can be cut 20% by judicious paring of "nonessential" items. Making deductibles and copayments average out at 80% each cuts another 36% off the rate to be charged. Another 10% can be cut off the rate by charging token amounts for office visits and house calls. These cuts alone when multiplied together bring prepayment rates down to less than 50% of the total per capita cost.

Other reductions for the typical family are made by charging a special family rate that is less than the sum of the single rates that families would otherwise pay—a strategem that increases the rate for single persons who are supposed to be able to afford it. Also, the rate for typical families can be eased down by charging elderly groups, like medicare members and other high user groups, special rates to compensate for their greater use of health services.

Other variations in payment plans involve use or nonuse of fiscal intermediaries. Large health care establishments merchandise their plans, assume the risks, and collect the premiums. But most centers use intermediaries for these functions. The different kinds of intermediary arrangements are listed below.

Functions Performed by Intermediary:

SALES:	Yes, No.
COLLECTIONS:	Yes, No.
RISK TAKING:	All, Some, None.
REMITTANCE METHOD:	Straight Modified Fee For Capitation, Capitation, Service

Prepayment plans are merchandized by insurance companies including the Blues, which are experimenting with HMOs. They make collections, assume part of the risk, and remit on a modified capitation basis. They could assume all of the risk and remit on a fee-for-service basis, or assume none of the risk and pay straight capitation.

The prevailing practice is for the carrier to assume the risk of catastrophic cases. Some carriers will also underwrite part of the losses a center suffers in a bad year.

Under the federal blueprint for HMOs, modified capitation is prescribed. HMOs are allowed to reinsure for catastrophic cases of $5,000 or more per year. They can also reinsure for reimbursement of 90% of costs in a single year that exceed 115% of revenues.

While possible prepayment plans are numerous, plans available to a given practice are restricted to a few by practical considerations. Establishments of less than 50 practitioners need a carrier to underwrite their plans, and carriers are not readily available to everyone who wants them. Carriers that can be interested in a given group will dictate terms of the payment plan. This situation will probably change in the next few years so that care centers will have a choice. For those that have some say in the matter now, or in the future, the following criteria might be considered in selecting a prepayment plan.

1. Make the plan competitive in price by limiting the care package to essentials and proven items of preventive care, by deductibles, copayments, and add-ons.
2. Meet competition on special family rates.
3. Charge extra premiums for the high use classes, but not to exceed the extra costs incurred.
4. Consider doing without a carrier intermediary if your center has 50,000 or more enrollees.
5. Employ intermediaries to assume all or part of your risks if you are a small or medium-sized clinic.

Practitioner Reimbursement Alternatives

About one-half of Horace Cotton's book, *Medical Group Practice*, is devoted to compensation of practitioners and for good reason. Nothing can destroy a group faster than an inappropriate reimbursement plan. The reimbursement arrangements for practitioners fall into three general classes, those applying to: large integrated establishments; small integrated establishments; and federated establishments.

Integrated establishments large enough for a hierarchy of practitioners have compensation plans like those in other large industries. The generic structure of these plans is suited to hierarchical organization. An astute observer can find variations within their common configuration but the common features are so prominent they give the impression that all such plans are alike.

The hierarchical plans are tied to job structure. Job status is the main criterion for evaluation. Base salary ranges exist to which each job is related. Jobs are assigned within the salary ranges in accordance with hierarchical position, give or take some weightings for differences among specialties. A hierarchy might include the following levels:

- National medical director
- Regional medical director
- Divisional medical director
- Chief of staff
- Department head
- Staff physician
- Resident.

One plan differs from another in how jobs are structured and length of the pecking order. Differences involve the structuring of salary ranges, how they relate amount-wise from level to level and how they overlap with one another. Methods used in job evaluation account for other differences.

Most plans relate jobs to one another internally. They also relate internal jobs to external ones by key jobs common both to the inside and outside; salary levels are adjusted by the key jobs. They are used as yardsticks to measure external salary increases and to convert them to commensurate internal increases. By this means, most administrators keep inhouse job rates competitive with industry scales.

Under the hierarchical approach, physicians get more pay by getting promoted and by general salary increases. In most plans, they can also receive merit increases for excellence or long service, but increases are limited by pay ranges of job category.

Enterprises provide performance incentives. Some use group incentives; others individual incentives. Physicians often share profits, some on a flat per capita basis, others as a percentage of base earnings. In HMOs, physicians must share capitation losses as well as gains. Individual incentives are usually based on physician contribution to gross or net revenues. Centers often keep detailed records of revenue generated by each physician, and in cases of measuring net revenues, the expenses of each.

Small integrated establisments usually have pay structures based on jobs, but the plans are not as formidable as those in larger organizations. Also, factors other than job content are stressed, such as seniority, reputations, and patient following. Often a point system is used with weights for each attribute. The points are calculated for each doctor. Shares of proceeds are determined from the point scores.

The federated groups, which are made up of quasi-autonomous units, nearly always adopt a system of compensation that corresponds as closely as possible to what the situation would be if all its units were truly independent. Separable revenues and expenditures are distributed to the units responsible for them, common revenues and expenditures are distributed in accordance with sharing formulas.

In the groups that keep records on individual performance, codes are used to identify services rendered. Often they use the American Medical Association procedural codes — generally with modifications to suit specific situations. Sometimes point values are awarded for each service rendered, for which many clinics use the California Relative Value Scales.

The proper generic pay plan for an establishment is fairly well determined by its organization type. Big integrated organizations require the highly structured plans that tie into organization hierarchy. The smaller integrated groups require simpler and more personalized systems. Federated groups require systems that are nearly autonomous.

Variations within generic plans pose alternative choices difficult to make. Should salary ranges rise gradually or steeply as one goes up the organizational ladder? How much weight should be given to seniority versus performance?

We suggest the following guidelines to fashion compensation methods:

1. Adopt the generic type customarily used by cognate enterprises.
2. Make the plan simple to understand.
3. Keep it flexible.
4. Adjust it to changing conditions.
5. Formalize the plan.
6. Keep records of individual practitioner performance to justify the plan as required.

Point 6 is the most critical and least honored. Compensation methods are always being attacked. If a method cannot be adequately defended or altered to meet legitimate complaints, it will harm the group, if not destroy it. The best antidote for attacks is performance information that reflects how dissident practitioners might make out on their own.

Fringe Benefit Alternatives

Fringe benefits are a part of the total compensation package. They consist of the things that an enterprise buys for its personnel, either because it has to by law, or because of the economy of buying in bulk, and most important, because it can save income taxes for its staff. For example, a head of a household getting a $15,000 package including $5,000 in benefits saves more than $1,000 in taxes yearly; another head of a household getting a $50,000 package with $15,000 benefits saves around $7,000.

Thanks to federal tax practice, fringe benefits are becoming a way of life. The term *fringe* is becoming a standing joke, but funny or not, benefit programs or the lack of them are making and breaking enterprises.

A menu of tax-exempt benefits and their costs as a percent of base earnings is shown in Table 6-7.

TABLE 6-7
Tax-Exempt Fringe
Benefits and Costs

Items	% Of Base Earnings
1. Retirement programs	2 - 25
2. Social Security — establishment share	3 - 5
3. Medical and dental insurance	3 - 6
4. Life insurance	0 - 2
5. Disability insurance	1 - 2
6. Unemployment insurance	1 - 3
7. Other benefits	0 - 17
Total	10 - 60

Another 10% of fringe benefits which is not included because it is not tax-exempt is time off for illness, vacation, holidays, and other reasons. Including both tax-exempt and nonexempt items, fringe benefits range in cost from 20% to 70% of base earnings; and the trend to higher percentages is continuing, suggesting a time when fringes will be larger than base earnings.

The other benefits category includes many new items, not in the main list, but shown in Table 6-8.

TABLE 6-8
Other Tax-Exempt
Benefits and Costs

	Items	% Of Base Earnings
A.	Company cars	0 - 5
B.	Meals on the job	0 - 3
C.	Other transportation	0 - 2
D.	Health services	0 - 2
E.	Recreation	0 - 2
F.	Education	0 - 2
G.	Professional services	0 - 1
	Total	0 - 17

There are more and the list is growing. According to lawyer Paul Techner in a paper on tax deduction published by *Physician's Management*, a fringe benefit can get tax-exempt status if the expenditure is adopted for good business reasons. The exemption plan must be properly documented and records should be kept to demonstrate how it benefits the organizational entity as distinguished from its individual members.

Benefit plans have limitations. Not all employees want all the benefits in their plans. Yet many enterprises insist that employees participate in all or most of the programs offered. This is resented by those who have to "pay in lower wages" for things they don't want. Even those who recognize the bargains they get in some of the bigger programs find themselves cash poor after tax and fringe deductions. One employee in a progressive organization expresses it this way: "I'm poor now but I'll be the richest man in the cemetery."

A good strategy for selecting a package of benefits is outlined as follows:

1. Keep abreast of benefits programs offered by other establishments.
2. Find out what the workforce wants.
3. Provide a basic package to include the mandatory and high demand items.
4. Enlarge the package as much as possible with elective items.

5. Consider the legal organization that gives the best tax exemptions.

6. Get professional advice from an employee benefit consultant or a legal firm specializing in benefit programs.

Item 4 needs emphasis. Progressive enterprises are considering "cafeteria style benefits." Each beneficiary would be allowed to make up his own benefits package from a menu of available items. Presumably each one would elect how much of his total compensation would be spent on benefits, up to a maximum, and would get the remainder in cash. The cafeteria concept has been partially adopted in that most plans have some elective features. It should develop more rapidly and eventually revamp existing programs and lead to new ones.

Capital Financing Alternatives

Considerable possibilities exist for financing startup, growth, and occasional realignment of groups. However, possibilities are one thing, getting capital is another. Sponsors soon find there are not as many opportunities as possibilities. Most of the time, they exhaust all sources of capital before getting what they need. So it is not so much a matter of having a choice of alternatives, but alternative sources from which to seek scarce capital. Few starting up enterprises can be particular, and some who have track records must scrounge for capital.

Often an enterprise has to change legal form to get capital. To get consumer support, a cooperative is needed. Employee capital can be obtained sometimes by creating employee owned groups. Grantors of funds insist on nonprofit status to get tax exemptions. Private investors want profit-making arrangements to get a piece of the action.

On the next page is a matrix (Table 6-9) that generates a range of financial structures.

For those who have a choice, there are combinations from which to choose. Some establishments, while taking what they can get at the start, gradually make over their financial structures to reach a chosen long range objective.

Some ground rules for those who have a choice are:

1. Stay independent enough to retain control.
2. Trade off some of the risk by attracting outside investors who have either a long range interest or special interest in the group.

TABLE 6-9
Financial Structure Matrix

OUTSIDE INVESTMENT:	All, Some, None
EQUITY INVESTMENT:	All, Some, None
COLLATERAL INVOLVED:	Much, Moderate Amount, Little, None
PATRONAGE INVOLVED:	
GRANT DOLLARS	Much, Moderate Amount, Little, None
GUARANTEES	Many, Moderate Number, Few, None
CREDITORS:	Suppliers, Staff, Patients, Employees, Financial Institutions, Individual Investors, Government
INSTRUMENTS:	Payables, Notes, Business Loans, Mortgages, Debentures, Preferred Stock, Common Stock

3. Borrow when interest rates are low; issue stock when they are high.
4. Avoid giving collateral when possible.
5. Accept grants as a last resort only, and only if they can be sanitized of undesirable strings.
6. Accept government loan guarantees only when needed or if they can be used to reduce interest rates 1.5% or more.
7. Borrow from the government only as the last resort.
8. Get a lawyer to review all new financing.

Thus, the possible ways of structuring groups are almost limitless. Opportunities, while a small fraction of the possibilities in a given situation, are also numerous, frequently overlooked, and often confusing by their number and complexity. They are treacherous because choice of inappropriate alternatives is often disastrous.

The job of choosing the right alternatives is an art. Guidelines exist, but they are crude and subject to continual refinement and revision. It takes people of talent to set the goals of an enterprise and reset them occasionally as conditions change. It also takes good professional assistance.

Setting goals is one job; attaining them is another. Not only does it take a high order of skills to create goals; it takes skillful planning and implementation to attain them. But that is an art in itself, and a subject for separate treatment.

Chapter 7
Development Planning
and Implementation

Every enterprise, including a medical practice, has two dynamic aspects: production operations and development operations. Production operations are the day-to-day activities that turn out products, usually in goods or services. Development involves change in the enterprise itself—its startup, growth, reconstruction, and so forth. Since the two kinds of operations are intricately woven together it is sometimes difficult to tell them apart. In a going concern, development is frequently sandwiched in with production; and frequently production people work on development projects. In fact, production people often contribute to development of an enterprise, even when they are working on production jobs—as when inventories or the flow of goods are built up in the development process.

One test to distinguish production from development is found in accounting. Operating statements reflect production; balance sheets through month to month changes show development. Of course, they both reflect only the monetary aspects of the two kinds of operations. But they do sum up in a common denominator the volume of each type of activity. To get these separate summaries accountants must single out and keep special records of development changes.

Health care enterprise development, then, is intricately related to service operations. Not only are development tasks interspersed with production, but they influence and are in turn influenced by service operations. Development changes in the last analysis are made to alter service operations, and changes in production levels often signal need for development changes of some kind, e.g., when clients are not adequately served.

The term *development* almost always connotes growth or betterment—perhaps because we are a growth minded people.

However, it can also refer to a decline. Some of the changes in an enterprise that development conveys are:

- Startup
- Expansion (routine)
- Major addition
- Improvement
- Contraction (routine)
- Spin-off
- Wrap-up

Outside of routine expansion and contraction of operations, which occur within a given production capability, the other items affect capability itself. They apply to projects that in some way change the capability of an enterprise.

While routine growth or contraction can take place within a given capability, it can often occur in projects that affect capability — such as when a new enterprise is created, and part of the job is to fill up the new pipeline with business. Sometimes this part of a project soaks up most of the funding allocated to it. The HMO Act, for example, allows nearly $4.0 million for creation of an HMO, and of this amount, $2.5 million is allocated to soak up operating losses during the initial buildup of operations.

Development processes have a common pattern whether they are applied to expansion or contraction. Although expansion means something is added, and contraction, that something is subtracted, the processes of planning and implementation for both are similar. Also, the processes used in both large and small projects are alike, except that small projects are less extensive and fall within the generic pattern of the larger ones. For these reasons, any development project can be inferred from description of a large encompassing one, such as the creation of an enterprise from scratch.

Today, public interest is focused on the buildup of practice, not on its cutback. And while it is true that only a few venturers start from scratch, they can easily relate their limited development to an encompassing pattern. Below are ten of the most prevalent kinds of projects, which fall within the encompassing generic pattern of a new enterprise project.

1. Creating a new enterprise.
2. Expanding a service line.
3. Acquiring new centers.
4. Creating new facilities.

5. Adding new support units.
6. Reorganizing.
7. Restructuring systems.
8. Revamping compensation plans.
9. Adding fringe benefits.
10. Installing control systems.

NEW ENTERPRISE PROJECTS

Though development projects of health enterprises have a common model, there are variations within the pattern. Some start from nothing at all and painstakingly build and assemble components to form final enterprises. Others put existing enterprises together: three solo practitioners combine practices; a partnership of two takes on a third practitioner, two groups of four giving limited care join to form a group of eight providing comprehensive care. The combinations are numerous. Few start from scratch; most build on existing practices — the logical and economical thing to do. Moreover, it is the ethical thing to do in neighborhoods that already have sufficient practices — unless, of course, the existing practices refuse to participate in a group venture that advances community health.

Starting from scratch takes a bundle of money. The practice has to be constructed before patients are recruited, and even with overlap of construction and recruitment, recruiting costs and startup losses are devastating in such ventures. HEW has encouraged creation of HMOs from scratch. The HMO Act supports this mode of development with liberal grants. HMOs can get the following amounts by grant or loan guarantee:

- Feasibility study $50,000
- Planning $125,000 (2 awards if required)
- Initial development $1,000,000
- Startup $2,500,000

Nearly $4.0 million per center is available. None of the amount is available for facilities, since HEW apparently relies on other capital sources for facilities, such as rental arrangement, purchase-leaseback, etc. If HEW were to finance facilities, another $4.0 million would be required for office care facilities, and an additional $8.0 million for inpatient facilities of sponsored HMOs.

A lot of new dollars go into HMOs. Only the government appears able to allocate this money, and it is getting "burned" in the process, as many new HMOs fail.

For those who can't get grants or don't want them, the logical way to create a CHO is to combine existing practices, which can be done for a small fraction of the capital required in the HMO formula. While capital used for tangible assets in this approach equals that of an HMO, total capital is much less since large startup losses that soak up capital are avoided. Our procedural descriptions are, therefore, based on building new enterprises out of existing practices rather than from scratch. It is not only the preferred approach but the dominant one as well.

Stages of Development

New enterprises are built up in two stages: a planning stage and an implementation stage. The planning stage can be conveniently re-divided into substages: an initial planning stage and an advanced planning stage. So in effect the two stages can be expanded to three.

- Initial planning stage.
- Advanced planning stage.
- Implementation stage.

The following scenarios describe the three stages.

Initial Planning Stage Scenario

A group of eight practitioners think they should form a clinic. They kick the subject around under an informal plan of periodically getting together until someone exclaims, "What the hell are we trying to do?" Then they consider whether to dissolve the group or get outside advice. They decide to get advice. An outsider comes in — possibly a consultant or lawyer — and suggests a feasibility study. It will cost $15,000. The study will define objectives, analyze them, state whether they are feasible, and give the economic prospects of the proposed clinic, including investment needed and future earnings expected.

Since $15,000 is to be raised and spent, it becomes time to incorporate. A for-profit corporation is created, officers elected, and a 1244 option executed so that if the project aborts within three years, the principals can deduct losses against their own personal incomes.[1]

A lawyer sets up the corporation for a minimal fee. He keeps its records in the early stages — if he knows simple accounting. Money is raised, the lawyer is paid, and consultants are hired to conduct a feasibility study. Several months later, they submit a report. If the report favors a new clinic, the amount of venture capital required is stated, and sources for getting capital are suggested.

At this point, the sponsoring physicians are somewhat shocked. About $400,000 of venture capital is required. Generally, everyone goes home when they hear the figure. In addition, it will cost another $15,000 to $25,000 to conduct a planning study, since the feasibility study is not detailed enough for prospective investors. The planning study will furnish an overall plan that can be used as a prospectus to raise the $400,000. Until the planning study is completed, the practitioners will have to foot the bill, or get a grant from the government. They take some solace from the 1244 option. At least they can get back through tax deductions nearly half of the $40,000 they might lose when the planning study is completed. The stakes are going up, but the game is getting more interesting. They decide to go ahead. At this point, the initial planning stage of the project is completed.

Advanced Planning Stage Scenario

The president of the new corporation calls in several consulting firms, gets bids, and decides to go with the firms that conducted the feasibility study because they need no indoctrination. A team of consultants enters the scene. They start with the feasibility study, review its findings, and become familiar with its backup data. They interview each principal at length, get his views on what is wanted, review each practice, and gather pertinent data on each, e.g., levels of operation, services rendered, systems, personnel employed, etc. They then review the neighborhood, look at census tracts, and make samplings to determine the likely market for health care services.

With this background, the consultants prepare policy guidelines for the new organization, checking them with the principals. They also formulate and check on the long-range objectives. Service lines are defined; a care package is designed; systems are predesigned, and equipment and other material needs are determined. Organization structure is drawn up. Key jobs are defined, and levels of operations are projected five years in advance. Staffing and space requirements are determined; building sites are designated; and facility specifications are roughed out.

Once these objectives have been approved, the consultants work up an implementation program. Steps necessary to achieve planned objectives are defined. They are woven into a program network, sometimes called PERT. Each task is described and scheduled. A project organization (an adjunct of the basic organization) is drawn up, and staff requirements are determined. The program is checked out with principals. Pro forma financial statements are prepared—operating statements, balance sheets, and cash flow statements for ten years in advance. Development costs are determined; startup losses are calculated up to a projected break even point. Capital requirements are then determined and scheduled.

The consulting team investigates sources of funding and makes exploratory overtures to potential investors. They select likely sources and prepare tentative prospectuses. The consultants submit their report with the advanced plan and bow out temporarily pending further work of others.

Lawyers and accountants enter. They draw up documentation for financing the venture. Principals solicit sources of finance, which may include themselves, since some of them may want a piece of the action. After considering alternatives, they settle on a private placement deal. It calls for creation of a service company that will own new facilities proposed, operate and maintain them, and provide administrative and technical support. Venture capital needed to do this amounting to $416,000 is pledged by a partnership that will get its money back in five years plus an equal amount in earnings and gains and the tax benefits of depreciation. As soon as financing arrangements are settled, the advanced planning phase of the project is completed.

Implementation Stage Scenario

An administrator is hired and given the job of implementing the development plan. Consultants are hired to assist him. A legal firm is retained to draw up contracts, and auditors are selected to review accounts. A construction firm is employed to draw up building plans.

The original venture corporation is converted to a service corporation, and the administrator is named president. The venture capital deal is completed. Temporary space is rented to house new administrative and support units until new facilities are ready.

A nonprofit corporation is created to be the core of the new enterprise. It will be the Plan Organization, that will handle medical plan functions and tie other units together. The new corporation is headed by one of the practitioners. In order to qualify as an HMO at some later time if desired, it elects sufficient consumer representatives to its board. It seeks essential public credentials, including a certificate-of-need.

The administrator, representing the Plan Organization, closes a deal with an insurance carrier who agrees to merchandise the medical package, provide reinsurance and collect premiums. A campaign is undertaken to sign up enrollees. Deals are closed with other providers: hospitals, extended care facilities and specialists.

Key personnel for the service corporation are recruited and indoctrinated. Contracts are drawn up for all major participants and key employees. Systems are designed in detail from predesign specifications. Individual practices and other providers join. New operations are started and superimposed on old ones.

At this point, the initial implementation phase ends and a shakedown phase begins. The new operations are built up as bugs are ironed out. Startup losses are analyzed and efforts are made to eliminate them. Compensation and fringe benefits packages are put into effect. Plans are completed for new facilities; financing for buildings and equipment is arranged. New construction is started. As new facilities are completed, operations are moved. Temporary space occupied by the service corporation is then released. Operations in the new facilities are expanded and improved until they begin to show a profit. At this point, the shakedown phase ends; the new enterprise is completed.

Development Similarities and Variations

The basic scenario has variation. For example, instead of being an independent company, the service unit might be provided by a supplier. Venture capital might be furnished by an insurance company instead of a private placement group. All along the line, one element after another might be replaced by another. But the overall pattern remains the same: each phase falls in sequence from initial planning to advanced planning and finally to implementation.

While the development process can be conveniently divided into phases labeled *planning* and *implementation*, each one contains both planning and implementation, since the two functions overlap. In fact, each major step that is accomplished involves six functions in the following sequence:

- Planning
- Preevaluation
- Decision
- Implementation
- Postevaluation
- Feedback.

For each phase, planning must be created—sometimes informally, at other times, more formally. Objectives are evaluated to see whether they are worth attaining, then a decision is made to go ahead or not. If the decision is to go, the plan is executed, and results are evaluated and reported back. It is a cycle that is repeated as the development process unfolds.

In the unfolding process, not all implementation takes the form of hardware. Much of it creates software or planning itself. In the so-called planning stages, the end product is largely documentation as general planning begets detailed planning in successive stages. The original scheme leads to the feasibility plan; it in turn leads to a development plan, and so forth. It is not until the so-called implementation stage that planning gets converted to hardware. At each stage in the development process, there is an external resource for what is needed. Lawyers provide contracts; consultants, the systems documentation; engineers, the building plans; and construction people, the facilities. For each item desired, there is a customary sequence that is followed — again, sometimes informally, sometimes formally.

Suppliers — whether they are inside or outside the establishment — are asked to bid on each job: what they can accomplish, how soon, and how much. Sometimes this is done in a formal request for quotation, or RFQ. More than one bid is often sought. Bids are made and submitted in proposals containing priced out plans of what each supplier intends to do. After the proposals are evaluated by the administrative staff, the suppliers are chosen. When a job is completed, the suppliers submit a statement or report of what was done. Often the report itself containing documentation of some kind is the end product of the task performed. All these steps have to be done meticulously with the appropriate degree of formality and detail, and in proper sequence. They constitute the development process.

BASIC KINDS OF PLANNING

The plan structure of a major project resembles a nesting hierarchy as shown in Figure 7-1. It starts with a general scheme reasonably well denoted but with meager detail. In successive stages of development, complete orders of detail are added at each stage, until enough documentation exists to complete the original scheme.

In the above scenario, the principals started with a general notion of what they wanted. By the end of the initial planning stage, they had translated the scheme into a priced out preliminary plan — the feasibility study. At the end of the second stage, they had a detailed development plan. During the implementation stage, they fashioned the documentation required — contract forms, specifications, layouts, diagrams, procedures, etc. Figure 7-1, incidentally, shows three plan structure levels; the number in the scenario was four (tentative scheme, preliminary plans, advanced plans and documentation). In complex programs there could be more levels — the number depends on the project's size and complexity.

FIGURE 7-1
Planning Hierarchy

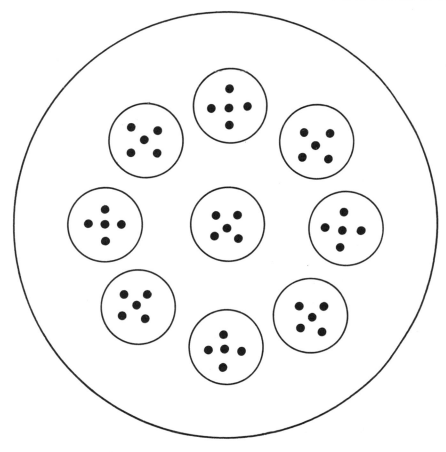

SYMBOL	REPRESENTS
Large Circle	Preliminary Plans
Small Circle	Advanced Plans
Dots	Implementation Documentation

A project is developed in this hierarchical manner, not only because it conforms with the way we think, but to provide a series of decision points that preclude going too far with a losing propostion. Except for documentation, each level of planning includes data to check out whether a project is worth continuing. Even at the beginning, a scheme isn't pursued unless intuitive estimates indicate it may have merit. At the feasibility stage—when only one order of detail is generated, costing relatively little—if the project doesn't evaluate well, it can be aborted without much loss. Another check point is reached at the advanced planning stage after a second order of detail is provided, when the project can still be aborted without substantial loss.

It is, therefore, important to properly stage the planning of a project, evaluating successive levels of detail before going on to the next level. In this way, risk is minimized, and fiascos are avoided.

Except for detailed documentation, a complete plan contains four major parts:

- Background information
- Objectives
- Program of execution
- Evaluation

The background information reveals the setting in which the project takes place. It describes the existing situation, the opportunities, and the constraints to seizing opportunities. Objectives reflect the situation to be attained. They are stated in just enough detail for the level of planning undertaken. Programs of execution state how objectives will be attained—steps to be taken, when, and who will be responsible for each step—in sufficient detail to accomodate the level of planning undertaken. Evaluation includes sufficient data to decide whether a project is feasible and worthwhile. Thus, the plan structure of an overall project is at best somewhat involved. It evolves in successive stages of detail, and each temporary culmination in the process provides a complete overall picture of what is wanted in greater detail than that of the prior stage.

Finally, the plan structure for the overall project is complicated by another order of plans—the plans for developing the overall plan itself. Not only do we have to create the overall plan in successive stages, but each stage in the process has to be planned. The feasibility study has to be planned, the advanced planning study has to be planned, etc. Plans for each stage of work are usually formulated in the proposals for conducting work on the overall plan.

The plan structure of a project is a key to its success. Plans must be structured properly to attain objectives when they are wanted and at the best possible cost. The plans need not be highly detailed as long as they are properly proportioned to suit each situation.

Overall Project Plan Example

To illustrate the parts of a plan, the following example — extracted from a real case, and simplified — is provided. The case involves eight practitioners serving 7,200 patients in a bedroom community sandwiched between two metropolitan areas on the East Coast. The practitioners are considering consolidating their practices to form a CHO. They have gone through the feasibility study stage and have just completed a development plan. Extracts from that plan with commentary follow.

Background Statement Example

Hamilton Medical Organization is located in Hamilton, New York, a city of 33,000 in 16 square miles of suburban countryside. It is a shell organization established to develop a comprehensive health care organization. Eight physicians serving 7,200 patients are involved. They are considering consolidating their practices.

Since most of the available land for residences is used up, city planners expect slow growth in the future. Today's median age, now 22, is expected to rise in a decade to 27. The population is largely middle-class, family-oriented, with less than a thousand medically needy people. About half the working population is blue collar, the other half is white collar.

At present only three physicians are in the community — a surgeon, an internist, and a GP. There are 23 physicians in surrounding communities, which have a combined population of 150,000. A distribution of physicians and providers in Hamilton and surrounding communities is shown in Table 7-2. Community hospitals close enough to serve the area are shown in Table 7-3.

Hamilton residents enjoy good health. A recent multiphasic screen of city employees, however, showed that only 45% were free of abnormalities, 13% had one abnormality, 33% had two, and 9% had more than two — indicating that apparent good health sometimes disguises asymptomatic incipient illness. A consultant's report to the mayor in 1973 showed that findings on the city employees were sufficient to conclude that the community might benefit significantly from preventive care. It was this report that prompted the physicians to consolidate.

FIGURE 7-2
Map of Hamilton, N.Y.

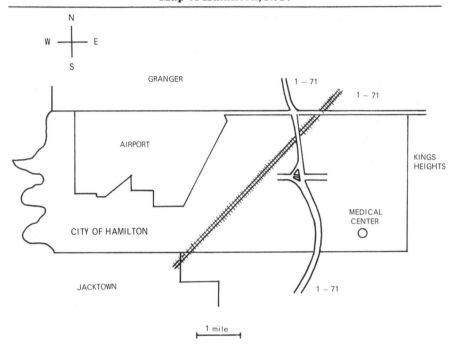

TABLE 7-1
Estimated Population (000s)
Hamilton, N.Y.

Population by age group	1975	1980
0 - 20	15	16
21 - 64	17	19
65 and over	1	1
Total	33	36

Counting long-term illness as one incidence, the number of illnesses in Hamilton during 1975 is shown in Table 7-4. Medical services delivered to the inhabitants of Hamilton and cost incurred for the year 1975 are shown in Table 7-5. A rough estimate of the cost of illness for the year 1975 amounts to $50,000,000. Table 7-6 shows the breakdown.

TABLE 7-2
Providers in Hamilton and Surrounding Areas

	Hamilton	Kinds	Jacktown	Granger
Internists	1*	4	2	
Ob/Gyn		2	1*	
Urologists			1	
Ophthalmologists			1	
Pediatricians		2*		
General Practitioners	1*	6	2*	
Surgeons	1*	2		
Dentists	2	6	6	6
Other Practitioners	1	3		
Pharmacies	2	3	1	6
Nursing Homes	1			4

*Designates the eight principals

TABLE 7-3
Hospitals in Hamilton and Surrounding Areas

Name	Community	Miles Away	Number of Beds
Southwest General	Kings Heights	8.0	180
Fairview General	Jacktown	5.0	150
St. Mary's General	Jacktown	8.5	100
Bay View	Granger	14.0	300

Many opportunities exist to improve medical services in Hamilton. Some of the services that are inadequate or lacking are: (1) an easily reached emergency center; (2) preventive medical care (periodic examinations, citywide immunization, and health education); (3) home health care; and (4) alcohol and drug abuse therapy.

The mayor and public-spirited citizens are interested in health care improvement. They want to attract more physicians who will provide

TABLE 7-4
Disorder Spells in Hamilton (1975)

Long-Term:		
Obesity		6,000
Tension, anxiety, and depression		3,000
Muscles, joints, and bone disorders		2,600
Heart disorder		2,000
Hypertension		1,900
Alcoholism		1,100
Diabetes		1,000
Other		4,400
	Total	22,000
Episodic:		
Acute illness		30,000
Treatable accidents		6,000
Pregnancies		1,000
Infant illnesses		4,000
	Total	41,000
	Grand Total	63,000

comprehensive care in modern facilities. They are willing to cooperate in related matters such as taxes, zoning restrictions, and other pertinent areas. Physicians of Hamilton Medical Organization see the opportunities and are eager to comply by creating a modern health center.

Objectives Example

The following tentative policy will be adopted by the newly proposed medical establishment, which will be called Hamilton Medical Park.

Policy of Hamilton Medical Park

1. To contribute to improvement of life quality in Hamilton through better health care.

TABLE 7-5
Health Services Delivered in Hamilton (1975)

Services	Number	Cost (000)
Deliveries	1,000	$ 750
Major surgery	600	750
Minor surgery	1,800	400
Physician visits	110,000	2,100
Dental visits	45,000	900
Drug prescriptions	120,000	900
Clinical tests (excl. hospital)	200,000	400
X-rays (excl. dental)	18,000	400
Short-term hospital days	34,000	3,600
ECF days	17,000	500
Other items		760
	Total	$12,000

TABLE 7-6
Estimated Cost of Illness
in Hamilton (1975)

Premature mortality		$11,000,000
Absenteeism due to illness		15,000,000
Incapacity		12,000,000
Cost treatment		12,000,000
	Total	$50,000,000

2. To make a high order of comprehensive health care available to the people of Hamilton by means of an efficient health care clinic.
3. The clinic will eventually serve up to 50% of the people in the community and will grow with the community.

4. It will attract and hold outstanding medical providers and will draw upon the resources of hospitals, nursing homes, and others to provide comprehensive care.

5. It will provide health care in pluralistic ways including services for fees and several kinds of prepaid care to keep patients well and to treat them when they are sick.

6. It will enroll patients without discrimination of any kind.

7. The clinic will be self-supporting.

8. It will charge competitive fees and premiums and will keep costs low enough to earn sufficient surpluses or profits for prudent expansion and improvement.

9. Control of the health plan functions and the organization that is responsible for them will remain in the hands of the practicing physicians.

10. Community spokesmen and others who might represent patients will serve as trustees of the health plan organization.

In cooperation with the city's mayor and other health care establishments, Hamilton Medical Park will strive to meet the goals listed in Table 7-7 by 1985. Other major goals of Hamilton Medical Park are shown in Table 7-8.

TABLE 7-7
City of Hamilton Health
Care Goals (1985)

| | | Costs in 1975 Dollars | |
		1975	1985
Premature mortality		$11,000,000	$ 8,000,000
Absenteeism		15,000,000	12,000,000
Inefficiency		12,000,000	10,000,000
Cost of treatment		12,000,000	12,000,000
	Total	$50,000,000	$42,000,000

Note: Population for '85 projected at 36,000 compared to 33,000 in '75.

TABLE 7-8
Major Goals of Hamilton
Medical Park

End of:	Goal
1976	Plan and organize Hamilton Medical Park.
1977	Begin new operations.
1978	Start new construction.
1979	Complete construction.
	Reach break even in operation.

The organization of Hamilton Medical Park is shown in Figure 7-3.

FIGURE 7-3
Proposed Organization for Hamilton Medical Park

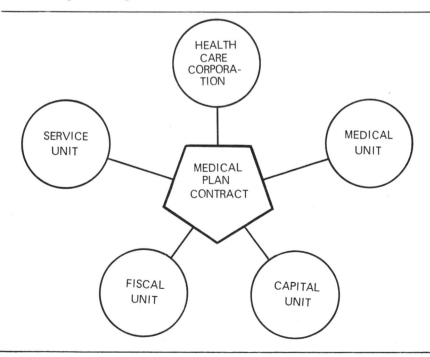

The health care corporation will tie the units together by a medical plan. It will provide patients with medical services acquired from physicians in the plan and from outside providers as needed. The medical unit with supporting services from other units of the center will take care of patients. The service unit will provide ancillary services including drug distribution, laboratory service, health education, emergency care, administrative support, etc. The fiscal unit will provide enrollees with health insurance, collect funds, reimburse providers, reinsure for catastrophe and other unusual needs, and maintain adequate cash reserves. The capital unit will supply funds for development, startup and working capital in return for capital fees commensurate with risks involved.

Table 7-9 shows the services that will be provided by Hamilton Medical Park, either inhouse or by outside subcontractors.

Hamilton Medical Park will include a 10,000 square foot modern medical building located near the residential center of the city, with parking space for 128 automobiles. Facilities will be flexible and expandable to 24,000 square feet.

TABLE 7-9

Proposed Services for Hamilton Medical Park

Primary Care	Medical Support	Other Support
Patient Education	Lab Services	Booking
Patient Health Audit	Diagnostic X-Ray	Billing
Physician Care of:	Pharmacy	Bookkeeping
Baby	Prosthetics	Scheduling
Mother	Medical Supplies	Reception
Others	Medical EDP	Other EDP
Dental Care	Staff Training	Other Training
Therapy:	Patient Logistics	Other Logistics
Physical	Medical Communications	Other Communications
Psychiatric		Purchasing
Immunization		Supply
Institutional Care		Building Operations
		Maintenance
		Business Service

Figure 7-4 represents a schematic chart of the proposed flow of services at Hamilton Medical Park. Reading from left to right one sees the flow of services from providers to patients. Reading back again from right to left one sees the flow of funds that pay for services rendered. The new establishment at the time of break even will employ thirty-nine people. The distribution is shown in Table 7-10.

FIGURE 7-4
Proposed Flow of Services and Funds At Hamilton Medical Park

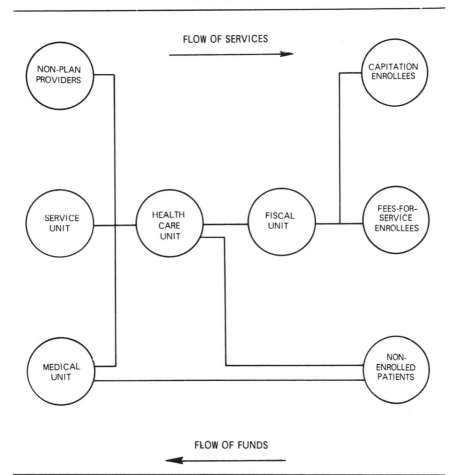

TABLE 7-10
Proposed Staff for Hamilton
Medical Park

Class of Personnel	Plan Unit	Medical Unit	Service Unit	Fiscal Unit	Total
Administrator	1/2		1/2		1
Medical practitioners		8			8
Medical support personnel		16			16
Pharmacists			2		2
Lab technicians			2		2
Educator			1		1
Insurance adjustor				1	1
Administrative support personnel			6	2	8
TOTAL	1/2	24	11 1/2	3	39

Evaluation Example

The proposed Hamilton Medical Park will start out with 7,200 patients and consolidated revenues of the eight participating practices amounting to close to $900,000 annually. In six years it will build up to $2,600,000 annually. In the beginning all of the units, except the medical groups, will run a planned deficit. By the end of three years, the operation as a whole will break even, and at the end of four years all of the units, except the nonprofit Health Plan Organization which will break even, will enjoy good earnings.

The matrix in Table 7-13 shows proposed income and outgo of funds through units of the new complex after it reaches full operations and starts to expand from 7,200 patients to half the population.

Patient revenues are anticipated to be $2,600,000 annually with $2,223,000 going to the intermediary from enrollees for service.

The intermediary getting $2,223,000 from enrollees will pay $2,111,000 to the health corporation for services to be paid for its own internal administrative services, leaving $21,000 from stockholders.

The health care corporation getting $2,111,000 from the intermediary for services to enrollees will also get $135,000 from the medical group and service company for rentals, making a total of $2,246,000. It will pay out $753,000 to the medical group, $494,000 to

FIGURE 7-5

Proposed Building for Hamilton Medical Park

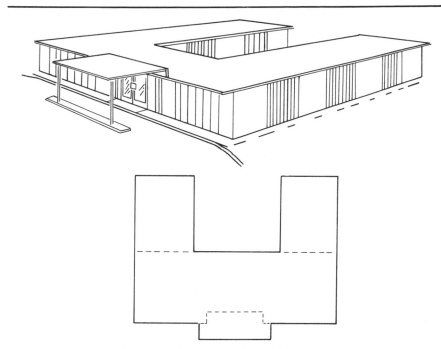

the service company, and $999,000 to others, respectively for services rendered to enrollees.

The medical group will take in $1,079,000, some $299,000 from nonenrollees, $753,000 from the health care corporation and $27,000 from the service company, respectively for services to enrollees. It will pay out the entire amount to staff and suppliers including $73,000 to the health corporation for rent.

The service unit will take in $572,000 with $78,000 coming from nonenrollees and $494,000 from the health corporation for enrollee services. It will pay out $62,000 to the health corporation for rent, $27,000 to the medical group for services, $438,000 to employees and suppliers, leaving $45,000 for investors.

Funds will be needed for working capital, software systems, equipment, and building until the proposed Hamilton Medical Park operation starts up, shakes down and reaches full capacity. Altogether $969,000 will be required, which will be collateralized with $416,000 venture capital.

TABLE 7-11
Hamilton Medical Park Project
Program Completed to Date

Events	Elapsed Time in Weeks		Doer	Profes-sional Man-Weeks
	Start	End		
Preliminary Exploration	1	4	Principals	—
Organize New Company	5	10	Consultants	1
Organize New Company			Lawyers	1
Feasibility Study	6	14	Consultants	6
Consideration & Approval	14	26	Principals	
Market & Resource Study	26	28	Consultants	4
Prepare Development Plan	28	32	Consultants	6
Investigate Financing	32	34	Consultants	2
Prepare Prospectus	34	38	Lawyers	3
Consideration & Approval	38	52	Investors	—

The Hamilton Medical Park Capital Group will put up the collateral and provide necessary financing. It will receive debentures and other negotiable instruments that will be repurchased by Hamilton Medical Park as cash becomes available over a six-year period. For taking the major financial risk, the Capital Group will be paid interest at commercial rates and a repurchase amount that will yield $410,000 for capital services.

A summary for the proposed financing is shown in Table 7-14. Thus, it will take $1,379,000 to develop proposed Hamilton Medical Park. The collateral risk will be $416,000; and the cost to raise that collateral will be $410,000 over a six-year period.

The investment will make it possible for the eight separate practices to combine and form a modern CHO that will improve health care in the community. The individual clinics that separately provide less than

TABLE 7-12
Hamilton Medical Park Project
Program for Completion in the Future

Events	Elapsed Time in Weeks		Doer	Professional Man-Weeks
	Start	End		
Realign Organization, Etc.	52	58	Consultants	6
Get Temporary Space	52	58	Principals	—
Recruit Key Staff People	52	66	Admin. People	—
Recruit Key Staff People			Consultants	4
Prepare Legal Documentation, Etc.	52	78	Lawyers	11
Contract with Providers	52	60	Principals	—
Design Systems	52	78	Consultants	26
Get Operating Funds	55	60	Admin. People	—
Contract with Intermediary	60	70	Admin. People	—
Contract with Intermediary			Lawyers	2
Contract with Intermediary			Consultants	2
Contract with Third Parties	65	75	Admin. People	—
Contract with Third Parties			Lawyers	4
Contract with Third Parties			Consultants	4
Recruit Subscribers	65	78	Admin. People	—
Recruit Subscribers			Consultants	12
Detail Organization	65	75	Consultants	4
Predesign Facilities	65	75	Engineers	15
Predesign Facilities			Consultants	4

TABLE 7-12
Continued

Events	Elapsed Time in Weeks		Doer	Professional Man-Weeks
	Start	End		
Negotiate Construction	70	75	Admin. People	—
Negotiate Construction			Consultants	2
Prepare Financial Plan	74	78	Consultants	4
Start up New Operations	75	130	Principals	—
Install Systems	78	114	Admin. People	—
Install Systems			Consultants	8
Recruit & Train Staff	78	114	Admin. People	—
Recruit & Train Staff			Consultants	8
Construct Facilities	78	114	Builders	—
Shakedown Operations	130	182	Admin. People	—
Shakedown Operations			Consultants	8

$1.0 million worth of health services yearly for 7,200 patients will increase their volume jointly to $2.6 million yearly. More capital equipment will be made available to each practitioner, and resulting economy will pay for the investment many times.

BASIC STYLES OF IMPLEMENTATION

Getting done what's planned is the name of the game. The best plans are useless if they aren't implemented — worse than useless if they go far astray. Each major stage of a project has its implementation phase, and each can go haywire. In the planning stages of a large project, implementation consists of converting general plans into detailed ones. The end product is often relatively intangible and difficult to identify. Jobs at these stages are frequently fudged when there is a lack of good follow-up.

In the implementation stage, the end product is usually both software and hardware. While only the software is susceptible to fudging,

TABLE 7-13
Hamilton Medical Park
Proposed Flow of Funds (Thousands of 1975 $s Annually)
7200 Patients

TO			FROM			TO
	Payers	Intermediary	Health Plan Corp	Medical Group	Service Company	Totals
Fiscal intermediary	$2,223					2,223
Health corporation		2,111		73	62	2,246
Medical group	299		753		27	1,079
Service company	78		494			572
Outside providers			775			775
Personnel		65	26	954	260	1,305
Suppliers & others		26	198	52	178	454
Investors		21			45	66
FROM TOTALS	$2,600	2,223	2,246	1,079	572	8,720

the hardware projects can get badly fouled up due to faulty coordination and confusion about who is in charge. Hardware changes are not only costly in themselves but almost always involve costly interference with production operations.

Overriding authority can be given to the project team. In such cases, a project manager is chosen and his organization is given line authority over all those involved in implementation. He virtually takes over and gets the job done. Wherever he runs into interference, the others yield. In contrast, the project manager is sometimes given only coordinating authority. He must sell the other managers on what needs to be done in their respective areas rather than order them around. Both extremes exist, but generally a hybrid approach is followed. Ideally, the project manager should be someone who has little line authority but can get what he wants done by leadership and persuasion. However, in the latter phase of a project, where signficant hardware is involved, it is often desirable to give the project manager strong authority.

Construction work needs strong direction because it often has to be done in the midst of day-to-day operations. Two general approaches

TABLE 7-14
Hamilton Medical Park Capital Group
Proposed Input and Payout of Funds
($000s)

Items			Years				Total
	1	2	3	4	5	6	
Input From Capital Group							
Working Capital	$130						$ 130
Systems & Organization	215						215
Equipment		104					104
Building		520					520
TOTAL	245	624					969
Payout To Capital Group							
Working Capital						247	247
Systems & Organization		70	75	82	88	94	409
Equipment		9	10	10	12	88	129
Building		7	8	8	9	562	594
TOTAL		86	93	100	109	991	1,379

are used. A project engineer with a clerk-of-the-works coordinates a federated group of outside contractors — masons, carpenters, pipefitters, etc. This is known as the conventional approach. The other approach is a turnkey job where one general contractor handles the whole thing. Turnkey jobs are getting more popular because they are easier to control. If done properly, however, the conventional approach can be cheaper since the lowest bidder of each class of contractors is employed. Construction can be done all at once or in sequential phases. In the Hamilton case, temporary facilities were contemplated while the new facility was being built. This had the advantage of getting the job done quickly with a minimum of interference in day-to-day activities. But, the Hamilton approach required a costly temporary setup and a subsequent move.

Sometimes it pays to sequence the construction program in two or three distinct phases. A modular building structure is adopted so that sections and wings may be added as time goes on. This approach is especially good when it takes time to develop an expanding market since capacity can be tailored to meet needs only as they arise, obviating a costly excess capacity.

Another variation in implementation style is the give-and-take allowed between planning and execution. Some projects are planned in the minutest detail, and implementation is held strictly to the letter of each planning document. Others are loosely planned, and project managers have wide discretion — even the authority to augment and replan as they see fit. Both styles have their places. In unique projects, the loose style often works best, while the stricter approach lends itself to repetitive projects.

The amount of outside help used is a variable factor. Some establishments prefer the do-it-yourself approach. Others rely heavily on outside specialists. When there is available inside talent, it should be used. But nothing can be more self-defeating than a project that is improperly staffed.

The best style of implementation to adopt is the one that gets the job done properly at the lowest cost. While strict conformance with blueprints is not always necessary, conformance with basic objectives and quality standards is. Time and cost schedules should be met, interference with production operations should be kept to a minimum, and idle time should be studiously avoided. To accomplish all this, a good follow-up system should be installed. Progress and status records should be kept, periodic reports compiled, deficiencies noted, and corrective action taken.

A rough set of guidelines for styling the implementation of a project is presented below:

- Appoint a well-qualified project manager.
- Make him responsible for the project.
- Grant him sufficient authority to get the job done.
- Give him discretion and a procedure for departing from detail specifications.
- Provide him with adequate staffing, allowing him to go outside if necessary.

Project work is an art practiced by people who specialize in it. It is essential that it be performed by those who are thoroughly familiar with the work.

NOTE

1. Sometimes lawyers forget a 1244 option which could be costly, as much of the initial investment in a losing venture can be recaptured as tax deductions. With the option, for example, the after tax cost of an unfavorable feasibility study is reduced from $15,000 to $8,000 or less.

Chapter 8
Aids and Sources

With the growing demand for improved health care has come the expansion of both actual and potential capability. The growth of actual capability shows up mainly in expansion of group practice. New groups are formed, and existing ones expand both in size and scope. This growth is rooted in one of the tidal movements — the industrialization of the medical industry. It is a manifestation of industrialization, a result of it, and a cause of it. By joining in groups, practitioners form systems of care that are streamlined, mechanized, and to some extent automated. New computer configurations help them to do this without sacrificing professionalism, decision autonomy, or the physician-patient relationship.

The opportunities of industrialization are attracting more physicians to group practice; this growth of groups in turn is inducing more suppliers to provide more resources for further industrialization. A stochastic evolvement takes place: industrialization feeds on itself to develop practices from embryo groups to mature CHOs. In addition to actual growth, the industrial process has enlarged the potential to expand group practice. Even though group practice grows rapidly, only a fraction of its full potential had been realized. The environment in which it develops is rich with opportunities and resources, which means that more growth is likely.

The resources for group practice not only exist but are relatively easy to attain. For practitioners who can perform professional duties, all other resources for developing and operating a clinic are available in the industrial market. There are roadblocks, it is true, such as government regulations, community rivalries, and traditional reluctance of people to make decision. But resources are there. What it takes to get them is ingenuity. In fact, one of the biggest challenges in

163

group practice development is to make intelligent choices among competing aids and sources of aid.

Potential medical capability is in fact, expanding faster than it is seized. Industrial suppliers are innovating vigorously, developing products for the medical industry, as they see the opportunities. As CHOs evolve, problems emerge and their solutions are not only critical to growth of the industry, but their possible solutions are opportunities for innovation with substantial market potential.

RESOURCES AND SUPPLIERS

As long as the principals of a group provide primary health care in-house, they can develop and operate a health enterprise by acquiring everything else from the outside. Moreover, they can do this even within the narrow HMO blueprint if they wish. The services of medical specialists, hospitals, nursing homes, therapists, optometrists, dentists and others can be obtained by prearrangements, by informal agreements or by more formal joint ventures that integrate specialists with primary care providers. This situation has been going on for some time. Group practices of generalists are successfully referring patients to specialists within the medical industry; and practitioners have joint ventured for years.

What is relatively new, however, is that *all* nonmedical services can readily be acquired in a variety of ways from several kinds of sources. Entire clinics and major support units can be leased; an encompassing number of end-item services can be purchased; and all the elemental resources for creating and operating a clinic can be conveniently acquired.

In fact, the resources needed to operate a clinic come in three stages of completion:

- Fully processed products and services
- Captive resource units
- Basic resources and raw materials

Fully processed products and services include end-items such as drugs, specialty care and health testing. Captive resources units include labs, pharmacies, and other units that turn out end items and intermediate products. Basic resources and raw materials include services, equipment, and other items that support inhouse service operations and the development of a clinic.

Fully Processed Products and Services

For each full-time-equivalent, primary care physician, totaling approximately 110,000, approximately $1,000,000 worth of care is given annually in the United States. Only 12% of the care is primary care; the remaining 88% is nonprimary care. So in a comprehensive care center consisting only of primary care physicians, the problem of acquiring nonprimary care for patients is paramount. Nevertheless, it can be done as most nonprimary care is available in fully processed form. Table 8-1 lists the fully processed items of nonprimary care, the potential yearly volume of each item per primary care physician, with some of the sources of care.

In addition to the $880,000 potential referrals, a primary care physician and his staff produce around $120,000 worth of services inhouse. In doing this, he relies on the outside marked for supply items. For each practitioner, these purchases amount to around $40,000 annually. Table 8-2 lists operating support items that are available on the outside, their volume per practitioner in dollars, and some of their sources. All told, 88% of the medical services rendered can be acquired from others. Of the remaining 12%, about one-third of the end-items can be purchased as partially processed supply items.

Captive Resource Units

All of the fully processed products and service items can be provided by captive resource units—in fact, everything including the services of primary care physicians can be acquired through such units. Table 8-3 shows the captive medical care units of a comprehensive health care group employing the full-time equivalent of ten primary care practitioners.

Nonmedical support services are also provided by captive units. Table 8-4 lists captive nonmedical service units for a group of ten primary care practitioners. It is predicated on staffing shown in Table 8-3, i.e., ten primary care physicians team with 20 other medical and dental practitioners and 74 technical service employees, but does not cover the captive hospital and nursing home shown in the table.

TABLE 8-1
Nonprimary Care and Suppliers
1976 Dollars

Nonprimary Care Items	Potential Yearly Volume Per Primary Care Practitioner $000s	Present Suppliers Nationally
Specialty medical care	$120	100,000 practicing medical specialists [e]
Hospital care (short-term)	400	5900 community hospitals
Nursing home care	55	800 qualified facilities
Dental care[a]	70	100,000 practicing dentists
Optometry	15	35,000 opticians, optometrists, and others
Other therapy [b]	15	30,000 chiropractitioners, podiatrists, and others
Drugs[b]	75	50,000 pharmacies
Prosthetics [c]	15	10,000 medical supply outlets
Radiological Diagnosis [b]	20	10,000 practices of radiologists [e]
Clinical Lab Testing[b]	30	12,000 private and hospital laboratories
Health Testing[d]	10	Several hundred centers
Dental Lab Work	10	8,000 dental labs
Fiscal Services	45	Several hundred carriers
TOTAL	$880	

[a] Excludes dental lab work.
[b] Excludes work in hospitals.
[c] Excludes optometry.
[d] Excludes clinical lab testing.
[e] Full time equivalent in active practice.

TABLE 8-2

Operating Support Services and Suppliers

1976 Dollars

Operating Support Items	Thousands of $s Yearly Per Practitioner	Suppliers Nationally
Facilities rental	$ 7.0	Several national companies REITs Thousands of real estate operators
Maintenance	1.0	Several national companies Thousands of local service dealers
Housekeeping Feeding Linen and laundry Ambulance service	1.0	Several national companies Thousands of local contractors Thousands of local, public and private units
Data processing	2.0	Several national companies Thousands of local units
Marketing and fiscal	10.0	Hundreds of carriers
Word processing	0.5	Thousands of local units
Investment counseling	0.5	Hundreds of national companies Thousands of local banks and others
Fringe benefit programs	25.0	Government Thousands of insurance companies and trusts
TOTAL	$40.0	

TABLE 8-3

Captive Medical Care Units of a

Ten-Primary Care Practitioner Practice

Captive Units	Size of Units
Primary care providers	10 Physicians[e] 10 Aides
Specialty providers	10 Physicians[e] 10 Aides
Dental care[a]	10 Dentists 5 Dental Assistants
Optometry	4 Employees
Other Therapy[b]	6 Employees
Pharmacy[b]	12 Employees
Prosthetics[c]	1 Employee
Radiology unit[b]	6 Employees
Clinical testing[b]	10 Employees
Health testing[d]	8 Employees
Dental lab work	2 Employees
Hospital (80 beds)	200 Employees
Nursing home care (50 beds)	50 Employees
TOTAL	354 People

[a] Excludes dental lab.
[b] Excludes hospital workers.
[c] Excludes optometry.
[d] Excludes clinical testing and x-ray processing.
[e] Full-time-equivalent.

TABLE 8-4

Captive Nonmedical Units and Sources of a Ten-Primary

Care Practitioner Practice

Practice Units	Size of Units
Entire Support Unit[a]	30 Employees
Operating Support Unit[b]	10 Employees
Administrative Support Unit[c]	10 Employees
Fiscal Support Unit[d]	10 Employees

[a] Includes the operating, administrative, and fiscal units listed underneath. Does not include professional and technical health care personnel or hospital and nursing home personnel.

[b] Includes clinical support operations such as transportation, supply, security, inhouse maintenance, etc.

[c] Includes administrative operations, such as booking, billing, bookkeeping, files, inhouse data processing, etc.

[d] Includes marketing, claims, collections, cash disbursements, income security, etc.

Basic Resources and Raw Materials

What can't be purchased in finished or semifinished form or obtained through captive units can be acquired in raw or basic form for subsequent processing into end-items. Practitioners can be hired, support personnel employed, and all other basic resources purchased. Table 8-5 lists the basic resources and sources for a ten-primary care practitioner, office-care-only practice.

TABLE 8-5

Basic Operating Resources and Sources

of a Ten-Primary Care Practitioner Clinic

1976 Dollars

Basic Operating Resource Items	$000s Annually	Work Force	Sources
Practitioners	1,500	30	Local community
Practitioner aides	300	24	Job market
Technical personnel	600	50	Job market
Building operation personnel	100	10	Job market
Fiscal personnel	150	10	Job market
Administrative support personnel	150	10	Job market
Drugs	300		Drug companies
Lab supplies	100		Supply houses
Prosthetic appliances	100		Supply houses
Medical supplies	100		Supply houses
Other supplies and misc.	100		Supply houses
Utilities	100		Tel., power co., etc.
Insurance[a]	600		Carriers
Fringe benefits[b]	800		Trusts, insurance companies, etc.
Property and income taxes	100		Government
Depreciation	100		Investors
Interest	100		Investors
Earnings	100		Investors
TOTAL	$5,400	134 People	

[a] Malpractice, income risk, property, liability, etc.

[b] Includes health, life, and disability insurance; disability and unemployment taxes; and employer-paid social security taxes.

In addition to the operational resources, most of the basic resources for creating and developing a clinic can be purchased. Table 8-6 gives a list of purchasable items with their sources for creation of one like that in Table 8-5 where 30 medical and dental practitioners are involved.

TABLE 8-6
Basic Development Resources and Sources —
Ten-Primary Care Practitioner Clinic
1976 Dollars

Basic Development Resource Items	One-Time Costs $000s	Sources
Feasibility study	10	Thousands of consulting firms
Planning study	25	,,
Legal organization, registrations and permits	15	Thousands of legal firms
Contracts and opinions	25	,,
Systems design	40	Thousands of consulting firms
Organization work	40	,,
Installation, training, and guidance	85	,,
Equipment	800	Thousands of suppliers
Building predesign	30	Thousands of contractors
Construction	1,200	,,
Land	300	Local real estate agents
TOTAL	$2,570	

Large sums of money are required to buy the basic resources for starting a clinic. In addition, working capital is required for day-to-day operations, and start up capital is needed to cover operating losses during shakedown. After shakedown, if a clinic is soundly conceived and developed, revenues will be sufficient to meet all costs and, in addition, provide enough surplus or profits to finance normal growth.

Table 8-7 shows sums of money, and their sources, for creation of a new comprehensive, ten-primary care practitioner, office-care-only practice (as in previous examples). It is assumed the clinic is created by consolidating existing practices.

Nothing turns off a group of sponsors more quickly than consideration of money. Millions of dollars are needed to create a large clinic. In the case illustrated in Table 8-7 more than $100,000 per practitioner is needed—and this amount includes nothing for inpatient facilities, and a minimal amount for start-up losses since it is assumed that existing practices are combined.

Much of the investment in the illustration is for working capital— assumed to be $1,000,000. It is needed as a cushion in paying outside providers some $4,600,000 yearly as well as inside costs of $5,400,000. The $1,000,000 of working capital is about five weeks of expenditure needed for seasonal fluctuations in payments, account delinquencies, and other cash flow variations. Most, if not all of the amount, can be obtained by pooling the working capital of practices consolidated and by prepayments of enrollees. The remainder can be staked by insurance companies handling prepayment plans, by banks, and by factoring houses.

Much of the equipment required for starting a new clinic is available in the practices consolidated. Generally, common use items such as lab apparatus and computer gear need be purchased. Most, if not all, of equipment investment can be raised by consolidating the equipment of principals, by bank loans, leases, and the installment credit of suppliers. Down payment for common equipment that may be needed can often be raised by sale and leaseback of the equipment consolidated in merging.

Consolidated land and building of merged practices, if available, can fill all, or part of, investment needs for housing new operations. If not, financial institutions may put up 75% to 90% of amounts needed. Mortgage loan guarantees are available under FHA, but there are many strings and red tape attached to them.

Guarantees are for 90% of a mortgage, which can save a percent or two on interest charges, reduce down payment needed from 10% to

TABLE 8-7
Financial Resources and Sources —
Ten-Primary Care Practitioner Clinic
1976 Dollars

Development Items	Required Investment $000s	Sources
Working capital	1,000[a]	Prepayments of patients. Principals' former receivables. Fiscal intermediaries. Banks. Factoring houses.
Equipment	800	Principals' former practices. Banks. Leasing companies. Suppliers.
Building	1,500	Principals' former practices. Banks. Savings and loan associations. Insurance companies. REITs.
Facilities Loan collateral, Development, and Start Up Costs	700	Private sources. Security markets. Insurance companies. Grants - federal - local - private SBICs. Consumers and suppliers. Government loans.
TOTAL	4,000	

[a] Includes working capital for paying outside providers such as specialists, hospitals, nursing homes, etc. as well as the sources serving the office practice only. The practice assumed in the table includes 30 practitioners, all told, serving 20,000 enrollees at a cost of $10,000,000 annually.

20%, or both. The working rule seems to be that it is worth paying an extra point of interest or putting down 10% more to be free of restrictions in loan guarantees. Where cash is short, however, a loan guarantee can make a venture possible.

The cruncher in financing is the last item in Table 8-7: the venture capital needed. Just as finance is the key to a new clinic, venture capital is the key to finance. It is the last 20% to 40% that is difficult to raise. This is the risk capital, the amounts that go for intangible things such as planning and shakedown expenses, and for down payments on facilities. Venture capital is what is lost if the venture does not turn out well; all the other capital is well secured. Consequently, few are willing to rush forth with high-risk venture capital unless they can make something of a "killing" in the event of success.

Not counting working capital, which can generally be raised when successful practices are merged, venture capital amounts to 20% to 40% of the capital needed to create a clinic. In the example in Table 8-7, it amounts to 23% of total capital, excluding working capital. In a smaller clinic, one of eight to ten practitioners, for example, venture capital is about 40% of the total.

Venture capital is "available" in many places—but the word "available" requires qualification. For promising ventures, venture capital is relatively easy to get, even in hard times. A promising venture, for example, might include consolidation of eight to ten highly successful practices—with the following features:

- Principals have good track records.
- Practitioners can work together.
- Business and administrative talent is available.
- Practitioners appreciate business problems.
- Good business prospects exist.
- A sound business plan is available.
- Practitioners participate in financing.
- Practitioners are committed to the practice.

There are two ways to get venture capital: one is through private investors, including the practitioners themselves; the other is by scrounging around for possible sources. According to a recent survey of *Physician's Management*, about 85% of clinic financing is made through private sources. Apparently, physicians do much of their own financing by making personal bank loans, often by putting up collateral to guarantee loans.

Other private investors often participate with practitioners in financing clinics. They seek a return on their capital commensurate with what they would get in other private ventures, and often take advantage of tax shelters in equipment and building investment. Private venturers not only want a good return but frequently insist on having practitioners take part of the action and make commitments that keep them from taking off if the going gets rough.

A few hundred centers have qualified in recent years for government grants and loan guarantees for which they had the obligation of becoming full-fledged HMOs. The Small Business Administration has guaranteed loans up to $300,000 for clinics, and SBICs have taken a stake in them. Insurance carriers have invested in quite a few "prototype" centers that are slated to become HMOs eligible for dual choice programs. Consumers such as companies and unions have financed centers, and suppliers such as drug companies have put up capital to create practices. Finally, some enterprising centers have gone into the securities market for capital—all the way from fancy underwritings to closely held intrastate issues.

Raising venture capital, especially through private channels, is somewhat sticky because of a prejudice against private venturing in medicine; and the more publicized the venture, the more likely it will be criticized. The argument that is put forth is that "people shouldn't profit from other people's illness." The cost of venture capital is about 2% of revenues for the first five years of a clinic's life. It is a small cost in terms of what it can bring about in better medical care. However, it does look large in terms of what the venturer puts up. But it must be remembered that the venturer is taking all the risk. If he didn't put up the capital, chances are no one else would. Moreover, clinics created by means of private venture capital apparently cost less to develop and have a much better chance of succeeding than those that are financed by government.

NEW OPPORTUNITIES

Although most resources for developing and operating clinics are available, it is still somewhat of a hassle to round up all the pieces. Suppliers have done a good job to date, but they haven't done a complete job. New kinds of insurance plans are needed to help clinics undertake comprehensive care without going the full HMO route. More and better ways to finance clinics are needed. There is also a need for support services by more companies in more comprehensive ways. More encompassing consulting services are required as is a center or place for interfacing the medical industry with other industry.

Insurance Industry Opportunities

According to the Health Insurance Institute in its 1976 *Source Book of Health Insurance Data*, the insurance industry just about supports the federal government across the board in programs to control the medical industry — PSRO, HMOs, HSAs, and certificates-of-need. Some consider such support a form of truckling, and well it might be, because many of the power centers with unusual influence in Congress have been beating the insurance industry for some time with the apparent objective of getting it out of the health insurance business. Thus, taking a strong pro government position may be a good defensive move. There are still some senators, such as Long and Ribicoff, familiar with the virtues of the insurance industry, who restrain the anti-insurance-company movement; and it doesn't hurt for the companies to take an "enlightened" position — even if it is against the wishes of the medical profession.

Not only does the industry support the government programs across the board, but it has been doing something about it. According to the same source book, "over 50 carriers have been involved in more than 70 HMO projects in over 25 states of which 21 are currently active." Also, the carriers provide reinsurance for HMOs and others to cover catastrophe, out-of-area, and stop-loss insurance.

The insurance companies have taken a bad rap for spiraling health care costs. It is the system, not the companies themselves, that has caused much of the inflation because no one is responsible for health costs. Physicians, patients, and other health care providers who make the decisions about use of services have no incentive to economize; in fact they have an incentive to overuse since the burden is distributed without penalizing individual overusers. Some public officials, apparently needing a scapegoat for the fallout of bad economic policy, have blamed the insurance companies for being lax with medical providers. This is done in spite of the fact that insurance companies have no authority over providers. They can set limits on what they will pay for a medical service, but they cannot dictate what fees will be any more than the government can dictate prices without price controls. This does not relieve them of the public beating they take, and it is small comfort for them to know that they are not responsible for every rise in insurance rates.

The insurance companies apparently see a way out of their uncomfortable position through development of HMOs. The HMO pins responsibility for medical costs on primary care physicians. Given just so much per head to keep people well, primary care physicians and their colleagues in an HMO must keep within a given overall budget or suffer the consequences in lower personal earnings. In HMOs it doesn't pay to overserve. It also presumably pays to keep enrollees well. In the perfect HMO, illness would be greatly reduced, cost of care would be less, and physicians could make out better than ever with less effort and strain. By creating HMOs for all care, it is reasoned, the current insurance system with its built-in inflationary tendencies would be replaced by a stable system that tends to hold down costs. This reasoning explains the enthusiasm among some insurance companies for prepaid care.

Unfortunately, the HMO prescription is not catching on rapidly. In spite of much support by government and insurance companies, the prescription is too narrow for widespread acceptance. Evidently insurance companies are not going to find the solution to their dilemma in HMOs.

While insurance companies cannot dictate fees to medical providers, they can help change the system by offering comprehensive care plans in which physicians undertake primary care of patients—much like they do in the HMO program, i.e., they can write insurance for care administered by physicians who agree to take on comprehensive patient care. Furthermore, they can merchandise such insurance among industrialists who are fed up with the continual increase in cost of conventional insurance plans.

Nor do the carriers have to follow the HMO prescription in devising such policies. In fact, it is essential that they do not restrict themselves too closely to the HMO formula, but that they broaden their approach to provide insurance for clinics that wish to develop along more liberal lines. For example, they can pay on a fee-for-service basis.

As long as responsibility for health management is pinned down to specific clinics, fee-for-service payments are feasible since clinics that get out of line costwise after consideration of patient mix and adjustment for catastrophe will simply bear higher insurance premiums. Deductibles and copayments can be devised without restriction in order to meet enrollees' needs and to encourage better consumption of care services. The care package can be tailored to provide the best mix of care and costs. In short, the insurance companies, together with users and payers of care, can develop a dual choice plan within the private sector to augment the one prescribed by the public sector. Other opportunities for insurance companies include:

1. Riders that will convert conventional policies to the health plans of CHOs.
2. Wider coverage of stop-loss insurance.
3. Financing CHOs that may not qualify as HMOs.
4. Provision of fiscal units to serve CHOs.

The administration of health care through CHOs opens up new approaches for carriers. Marketing and fiscal services, which are now centralized, might be conveniently decentralized. A CHO with ten primary care practitioners serving 20,000 patients and generating revenues of $10,000,000 — depending upon the marketing effort needed — requires an on-site fiscal unit of between five and ten people. In today's system, the fiscal cost amounts to a 8% to 10% override on the premiums charged — more than the $500,000 for the fiscal unit of five to ten needed in the ten-primary care practitioner clinic. It would appear that the percentage override under the new system might be reduced and still leave carriers with a profitable business. Moreover, a decentralized operation has other advantages: claims adjusters on the spot for preapproval as well as immediate postapproval of charges, and immediate processing of bills. In such a system, misunderstandings and long, costly disputes should be largely avoided.

Financial Opportunities

If present trends continue, a potential of 10,000 comprehensive care centers by 1985 is a distinct possibility. The development of such centers would take enormous resources — estimated at $30 to $40 billion for office practice operations only. Another $30 to $40 billion will be needed by hospitals and others for inpatient facilities to support CHOs. While there is overlap in the two figures (some hospitals will become CHOs) the total is estimated at around $70 billion in 1976 dollars. In inflated dollars, the total could exceed $100 billion. So even attainment of half the potential would require large sums of money.

Assuming the industry generates enough internally through depreciation, amortization and surpluses to finance $20 billion, it will need as much as $50 billion in 1976 dollars from outside sources. From

$10 to $15 billion of this amount could be in the form of venture capital, the remainder in the form of conventional financing such as mortgage loans, installment credit, and leaseback arrangements.

What is more interesting than the potential amounts to be put into the industry is the expected payout which is estimated at over $1.50 for every $1.00 that will be put in. It seems the industry on balance should be a generator of much investable capital. The chief reason for the anticipated favorable flow of funds is the pension and profit sharing funds that will be generated under new pension laws — $3 to $4 billion annually.

Finally, the industry as a whole is financially sound — in fact, one of the strongest in the nation. It is practically guaranteed 10% of the national income paid largely by financially strong industries and the federal government. Even without national health insurance, the amount that individuals pay out of their own pockets in the next decade will be less than 20% of the total national medical bill. For all intents and purposes, the industry is almost depression proof. In spite of widespread financial distress in both hospitals and municipalities in 1975, tax exempt hospital bonds sold well and accounted for the majority of hospital financing.

Yet, sponsors of new clinics must search for capital when they need it. Even though there are thousands of financing sources, it is not only difficult to find financing, but even hard to find out what is available. Financial people have overlooked to some extent the medical industry not only as a place of good investment but as a source of investable funds.

The key to investment opportunities is venture capital. Those who furnish venture capital to the industry have a jump on others, since recipients of venture capital are prone to make the more staple loans with the institutions that arrange for venture capital. Venture capital is not only the key to other opportunities, but profitable in its own right. A $400,000 investment in an eight-practitioner establishment can be rolled over in six years at a gain of 100% with attractive tax shelters for well-heeled investors. An SBIC or a large investment trust could do well with a carefully selected portfolio in health care establishments.

There is an acute need today for two or three investment centers in each metropolitan area and rural region specializing in health care financing. The investment centers could be operated by commercial banks with venture capital affiliations, by insurance companies, investment banking houses, venture capital affiliates of large corporations, and others. Such centers would work with health care institutions, developing and offering financial packages for establishments of all kinds and sizes. They would also develop and offer pension and other benefit packages involving the investment of funds. By filling this need, such centers might well prosper.

Service Company Opportunities

The business of providing service teams under contract is still in its infancy. A few companies provide such services in scattered parts of the country. Furthermore, the packages of services offered are usually limited to some functional items such as building operation and maintenance, housekeeping, security, feeding and administrative management. Very few outfits offer a broad spectrum of services.

The corporate hospital chains are providing physician suites in hospital settings in some parts of the country. They provide the space, building operations, maintenance, and some of the medical support services such as lab and pharmacy. Other hospitals are performing similar functions in varying degrees. Some of the investor-owned hospital companies are providing contract management to hospitals and large health care centers. They often provide capital for constructing facilities which they sell to a community and help manage. They also acquire health centers which they operate and leaseback. While this business is becoming significant, it is only getting started.

There is a need for more companies to provide service units in the health care field. Outside of finance, and possibly even eclipsing it as a roadblock, nothing stands in the way of clinic development as much as lack of medical support services and the talent to develop them. Even administrators and business managers are scarce, and good administrative support is scarcer. This need for support services presents an opportunity for enterprising companies that are skilled at providing captive service units to industry. A comprehensive health care center serving 20,000 enrollees needs a service support unit of 60 to 70 people, and a full-fledged unit is capable of generating $1,500,000 yearly. The potential market for such services in terms of 1976 dollars is $15 billion annually. A company fielding 100 units could conceivably gross $150,000,000 annually, which represents only 1% of the potential market.

Consulting Opportunities

Until recently, the medical industry has not been a heavy user of consulting services. Consultants are ready to concede that this is one of the reasons that business affairs in the medical industry tend to be backward. It is more likely, however, that delay in industrialization across the board has much to do with the sparing use of consultants. As the industry catches up in industrialization, its use of consultants increases. It is likely that in the next decade as CHOs are developed, the medical industry will become a heavy user of consulting services. Consulting firms that understand the business aspects of group practice and comprehensive health care are needed now, and that need seems destined to grow. Consultants are required to make feasibility studies, planning studies, do system design, perform organization work, search for key people, design benefit programs, conduct training programs, and consult on installation problems. These one-time chores generally are done best by consultants

At the same time, there is a shortage of consulting firms that understand the medical industry. Among those who do understand the industry, there is little standardization. Feasibility studies are done in many different ways, planning studies differ considerably depending on who does them, and so forth. Not only are the approaches to similar problems divergent, but fees charged for accomplishing similar objectives vary considerably. Evidently, the consulting fraternity through its several national organizations has a big job ahead to indoctrinate consultants in the medical industry and to adopt some consistency, if not standardization, in services performed.

The stakes ahead are big both for medicine and the consulting industry. In developing a CHO, there is need for several consulting man-years, worth about $150,000. It doesn't take many jobs of this kind to keep a good-sized consulting firm busy. In the next decade, the medical industry should be good for several billion dollars of consulting services, most of it to help develop health care centers. It is critical that these services be available and competently performed.

An unusual opportunity also exists for consulting firms that can help limited group practices convert to comprehensive care. The key to doing this economically is to establish an efficient health testing unit within a group practice. The cost of periodic health testing that is well balanced and comprehensive can be as low as $40 per person per year where volume is high and about $60 where volume is relatively low. However, these low costs can be attained only where a specialized testing unit is designed to suit the peculiarities of the clinic served. Health testing units come in a range of configurations—from $750,000 automated units good for 50,000 or more enrollees to $25,000 units good for several thousand enrollees. Consultants who come up with a planning technique to cover all conditions will have a jump on others in establishing CHOs.

Association Opportunities

Someone ought to create a medical-industrial association — someplace where medical people and industrialists can meet to explore their mutual problems. Such an association is long overdue, since the medical industry has become intricately involved with industrial equipment and techniques. About 40% of the dollars spent on health care yearly winds up in the coffers of other industry, and the amount now close to $50 billion annually is growing faster percentagewise than the cost of medical care, which in turn is growing faster percentagewise than the GNP.

Yet there is no permanent place or common center where medics and industrialists can go to learn from each other, to exhibit industrial products and hold seminars, to exchange information and to size up present markets and learn about new ones. It would be extremely beneficial if such a place existed.

As the momentum of change increases, the medical industry progressively seeks more aid from outside. Already the amount of outside aid is sizable and sources of aid are abundant. Since more will be needed, new opportunities await the resource suppliers of the industry. When the final account is written, it is likely that the emerging health care system will be largely the product of a massive interaction between medical groups and the suppliers of medical resources.

Chapter 9
Conclusion

The development of group practice is significantly changing the medical industry, if not revolutionizing it. Straight across the board there is a progressive grouping of physicians. Solo practitioners are either joining with one another to form two-man partnerships and groups, or are sharing space and other resources in informal arrangements. Two-man partnerships are expanding to form three-man groups, and most groups with three or more practitioners are enlarging both in numbers of practitioners and in numbers of patients. In addition, groups are enlarging their spans of practice. Some that formerly gave limited care are considering the practice of comprehensive care. HMOs, neighborhood health centers, and private versions of comprehensive health care centers are springing forth, many hospitals through outpatient units are giving a form of comprehensive care to an estimated 20 million or more patients, a number that is growing in large increments each year.

Group practice is the natural outgrowth of the industrialization of medicine. With the decline of contagious disease, largely made possible by the drug industry, doctors have been able to pull back from home-oriented practice to office practice. This has allowed them to congregate in medical centers such as downtown professional buildings, hospitals, and specially created clinics. It has allowed them to specialize and to develop streamlined handling processes, which together with fewer house calls has helped them double their output of services per physician in less than a generation. In addition, they have taken advantage of miracle equipment that extends their capability immensely; and through pooling of resources, they are able to use equipment that would otherwise be beyond their reach. Moreover, the accelerated demand for industrial products as physicians group together stimulates industrial innovation and growth—a process that apparently feeds on itself and is reaching a new highpoint every few years.

Federalization acts as another spur to group practice. Gradually government at all three levels is encroaching upon the practice of medicine; much of the federal program is oriented toward creation of group practice. A kind of carrot-and-stick policy is pursued — the government offers rewards to those who create group practice, and difficulties, if not penalties, for those who do not. Regulations are imposed on the industry which make it virtually impossible to practice without a staff of business experts that only groups can afford. But as an incentive to form groups the stick policy works in reverse, too. Many physicians are wary of groups simply because government and attendant bureaucratic spokesmen push them. In addition, since group practice "government-style" doesn't appeal to many solo practitioners, it tends to sour them on all group practice.

A third spur to group practice is the comprehensive care movement. Doctors are being called upon to keep people well, not only to treat them when they are sick. In the past the emphasis was to treat illness, and because of economic factors, routinely keeping people well was largely an ancillary duty, time and money permitting. In recent years, the medical industry has found ways to practice preventive medicine more effectively through analyzers, diagnostic equipment, and computers — products of industrialization as well as medical innovation. Slowly physicians have been adopting the new techniques to expand well-care. Government officials and the media, sensing a good thing several years ago, jumped on the bandwagon and pushed the concept of comprehensive care. Now it appears that the general public wants it faster than the medical industry is capable of giving it. The solution to this dilemma seems to be in group practice where comprehensive care can be given more economically than in solo practice.

So it appears that solo practice is doomed except for those medical superstars who are so rare that they can best serve by staying independent and on call by groups as they are needed. The rest of the solo practitioners will find their way into groups. In spite of the regressive features in federal programs, group practices are likely to grow until the medical industry has been truly reconstructed, probably in the next ten years.

The federal government has a blueprint for group practice: the HMO blueprint. It is surprisingly broad in some respects, and as regulations are issued, it gets broader. In fact, regulations have been broadened to the point where they call for new legislation. But even with the broadening, the HMO blueprint will still be too narrow for universal, or even encompassing acceptance.

There is a much broader blueprint which will accomplish those objectives of the HMO program that we consider desirable. The blueprint, while not a formal one, can be fashioned out of the experiences of successful groups in the country and the literature describing them. It not only encompasses the narrower HMO version but covers successful clinics that do not qualify today as HMOs. Under the broader CHO blueprint, featured in this handbook, doctors can create clinics that retain most of the desirable features of solo practice while acquiring the advantages of group practice. Moreover, the clinics established on the broader blueprint can do anything an HMO can do — probably more effectively — including control of costs so badly needed by the industry.

Most group practices in the future will probably be created under the broader blueprint for CHOs. Doctors apparently prefer it, and it could give industry an effective means to carry out the dual choice program of the HMO Act. While the government is trying to work the kinks out of HMOs, the private sector could develop its own kind of health care centers under the more acceptable CHO formula. It is even possible that by the time government gets through the HMO formula, it will resemble the CHO one.

Under the broader blueprint, all it really takes to create a group, according to the definition of a group, is to put three solo practices together, or to add one solo practice to a two-man parrtnership. The group can then become a CHO by adding a routine health testing function, patient education, an inoculation program, and an adequate patient record system. A convenient add-on, in addition, would be a prepayment plan which the group could either offer itself with insurance company backup, such as insurance for catastrophe and other unusual loss, or one which insurance companies could offer by riders to conventional policies or in other ways.

All of the resources for setting up group practices are available, and while insurance for prepayment is still being experimented with on a limited basis, it too, should be widely available in the near future. While there are a few roadblocks, it would appear that conditions are favorable for rapid development of group practice and for the conversion of limited group practices into CHOs.

As this is done, the question arises: Is it all worthwhile? What are the rewards, if any, in the evolving system of medical care? Strangely enough, there is no clearcut answer. The makers and shakers of the new system are largely going on faith. According to opinion polls, it is what the public wants—a dubious conclusion because the polls are ambiguous at best. Nevertheless, there have been no in-depth studies to indicate if the effort is worthwhile. There are extensive Congressional investigations, but these appear to be for the purpose of incorporating refinements in the current blueprint. Excerpts from hearings indicate that many medical practitioners think the government blueprint is no good. However, the power centers go on with their plans in spite of protest. They are evidently convinced they are on the right course for several reasons: they reason that something must be done about the present cost situation and that a new system that calls for group action in place of solo practice—one that stresses preventive care and contains incentives for providers—is bound to be an improvement. This belief together with some fragmentary information on industry economics, a favorable impression of the Kaiser plan, and notion that somehow we should copy our friends in Europe sustain many of the decisions that change our medical economy.

There are several reasons why we lack a clearcut answer to the question. First, the medical industry is complex and its phenomena difficult to define, which makes the economics of the industry unusually abstruse. Figures are plentiful, but few people can agree on what they mean. For example, one journal will put the incidence of hypertension at 10% of the population, another at 20%, because each defines the illness differently. This kind of apparent inconsistency pervades the industry. Furthermore, if one reconciles apparent inconsistencies, there is little time for anything else. The upshot is that nearly everyone freewheels medical statistics, adding to the general confusion. Another reason for the uncertainty is the absence of large and significant studies, perhaps because the power centers waited too long to consider constructive action. There have been few significant demonstration projects for the same reason. Since the Partnership for Health Act in 1966, HEW has conducted demonstration projects on a restricted formula basis, not sufficient to furnish answers to many questions that arise.

Thus, an answer to the question on worth of the proposed system must be forged out of pieces of information and reasoning. Our conclusion is a qualified prediction that the system will prove worthwhile if government and industry work together in good faith, with mutual respect, and in harmony. Concerning individual providers and sponsors, there is little question that rewards can be substantial for those who seize the opportunities.

THE PUBLIC GOOD

Whether the general public gets a good shake or not is the crucial question. In the final analysis, success will boil down to whether the system will pay for itself in the long run. The power centers are apparently gambling on substantial economic improvement. There are many statements being made that the system will give better health care at lower costs. Some less cautious prognosticators say it will give better care at the same cost; and a few foresee better care at a higher cost with resulting life enhancement outstripping the rise in cost. In all cases, the prediction is that the benefits-cost relationship will be improved. If this comes about, the new system will indeed be a success, and the power centers will have won their gamble. The general public will also benefit.

The critical factor which the architects count upon is preventive care. As many put it, preventive care should go a long way toward stamping out disease, extending life, and enhancing lifestyle. To make a case for this point of view, we assembled some facts and figures that are impressive, even though they have been taken out of reference books, magazine articles, and other sources, and, in the free-wheeling fashion mentioned, have been massaged for presentation.

According to numerous physicians, at any one time about one-half of the people in the United States have a physical disorder requiring medical attention now or in the near future. Some have more than one disorder, even three or four at one time such as the obese diabetic with heart trouble. In fact, if the disorders were spread evenly throughout the population, everyone would have at least one disorder at all times.

To better appreciate this, consider the statistics in Table 9-1. Notice that much illness is chronic, or slow in developing, with little or no apparent need for immediate medical attention. These disorders start as borderline cases, and depending upon definition, could be ruled out as disorders in the early stages. Some physicians might even exclude obesity and nervous tension as medical disorders, preferring to include mental disorder as a category, even though there is a correlation between obesity and early death, and nervous tension is a major eroder of physical well-being. The chronic diseases are often asymptomatic, i.e., they do not show up until advanced, and require preventive surveillance if they are to be discovered at an early time.

It is interesting to note that most of the disorders fall into a few categories. Even in the categroy listed as "Other," which masks such killers as cancer, nephritis, drug addiction, and serious mental

TABLE 9-1
Prevalence of Illness, 1976
(% of Total Population)

Chronic Disorders:		
Obesity		23%
Nervous Tension		10%
Muscle, joint and bone disorders		12%
Heart disorder		10%
Hypertension		9%
Alcoholism		5%
Diabetes		4%
Other		18%
	Sub Total	91%
Episodic Illness:		
Respiratory Infection		3%
Other		2%
	Sub Total	5%
	TOTAL	96%

Source: AJFCo Study

disorders, the great majority of cases fall into a relatively few sub-categories. Further, within major disease classes, such as heart trouble, which represents hundreds of disease species, one kind, myocardial infarction, accounts for most of the cases.

Physical disorder is the chief reason for our medical industry, which costs $130 billion annually. But it is not the only reason. As physicians will testify, there are people who think they are sick and demand medical care. Numbering up to 25% of the patient load, these people, according to some estimates, clutter the system, and physicians keep trying to weed them out.

A summary of the annual cost of medical services in the United States is shown in Table 9-2.

TABLE 9-2
Estimated Cost of
Medical Services, 1976

(Billions of 1976 Dollars)

Short-term hospital care	$ 45
Physician Services	26
Drugs[a]	8
Dental services[b]	8
Laboratory services[c]	4
Extended care facilities	6
Long-term hospital care	6
Other practitioners[a]	2
Prosthetic devices	3
Research	3
Construction	5
Education	1
Public health administration	4
Fiscal services	5
Other	4
TOTAL	$130

Note: [a] Excludes hospital share
[b] Excludes lab services
[c] Excludes hospital share and radiology
Source: Department of Commerce Data Extrapolated

While evidence indicates that the overall life span has relatively inflexible boundaries, the average has stretched a good deal over the years: from 49.2 years in 1900 to 71.2 years in 1971.[1] It appears that this longer life span comes from the elimination of premature deaths. Back in 1900 with life span below 50, almost all deaths were premature; while today premature deaths, approximately 40% of the total, are reaching tolerable levels. In 1900 the majority of deaths were caused by diseases that struck early as well as late in life; today the majority are caused by diseases that largely strike late in life.

Elimination of premature death would apparently increase present life span about 15%. It would postpone the deaths of some 800,000 people annually in the prime years of their lives, years when they are productive and needed. Furthermore, the possibility of substantially reducing premature death appears to be good. It is significant that most mortality today is caused by a few diseases which respond to preventive care: heart disease, cancer, and stroke, which account for nearly 70% of all deaths.

Physical disorders, in addition to causing premature death, are among the chief detractors of human happiness. About 50% of the population is handicapped healthwise to some degree, around 10% seriously. This takes its toll in grief, for which there is no price tag, and in productivity.

The significant conclusions are:

1. Disease and physical disorders apparently cost the American people around $360 billion annually: $130 billion for medical care, $145 billion for loss of human productivity, and $85 billion in premature death.

2. Relatively few types of disorders account for most of the economic loss and attendant grief.

3. A successful program of disease prevention could have a large pay-off economically.

The crux of this argument is in the last conclusion, namely that emphasis on preventive practice will pay off. With the available information no one can make an airtight case, but the trade-off possibilities look good. Potential savings in productivity and premature death — let alone the strictly human values — are in the order of $230 billion annually. With less than $10 billion annually now being spent on prevention, think what $20 billion on prevention might do.

An opposing viewpoint was expressed by Russell B. Roth, M.D., speaker of the American Medical Association House of Delegates, and reported in the *American Medical News* on March 27, 1972. Addressing the AMA's 25th National Conference on Rural Health, Roth told the assembled delegates it was arrant nonsense to expect either lower costs or improved quality from a system that requires physicians to emphasize preventive medicine. He went on to say, "Physicians today, in general, are trained to diagnose disease and disability and to treat them. Their mission in life is, almost by definition, one of sickness care."

Dr. Roth said further that preventive medicine does not promise substantial economy over the short or intermediate haul. To illustrate he asked his audience to take a hypothetical position that everyone should have an annual physical examination. With a price tag of $150 per examination, suggested by Dr. Roth, the total nationwide cost, according to his calculations, would be just under $31 billion a year. Other physicians put forth this argument which is, no doubt, convincing. Indeed, we have analyzed Dr. Roth's figures and find they hold up. We do not, however, agree with his conclusion that emphasis on preventive medicine is arrant nonsense. Dr. Roth did not comment on the benefits of preventive care; he merely emphasized its cost. But most important, in his hypothesis he assumed current practices and fees for giving annual examinations. With new approaches now being used, the old fashioned $150 physical examination is giving way to more effective procedures at less than $50 annually.

While it is true that physicians are not generally trained in preventive practice, we believe the time has come for a shift of emphasis. Doubling existing preventive efforts might increase the cost of care, but the resulting benefits could be enormous. For example, assume that expenditure on preventive care in a concerted effort were doubled and that the increased effort would cut down the prevalence of disease and the incidence of premature death by one-third. The comparative economic picture appears in Table 9-3.

PHYSICIANS' WELFARE

The public may gain; but what about physicians? For some physicians, the public gain would be enough reward even if they had to make sizable sacrifices to achieve it. With some doubt in mind that the public will gain, some physicians will be weighing possible disadvantages with other potential rewards.

Disadvantages to physicians are easy to visualize: the burdens of making major changes in practice from individual to group style with a shift in emphasis from curative to preventive medicine; increased

TABLE 9-3
Annual Cost of Disease Comparison
(Billions 1976 Dollars)

| ITEM | SYSTEM | | |
	Present	Proposed	SAVING
Cost of Care	$130	$140	$(10)
Loss of Productivity	145	97	48
Premature Death	85	58	27
TOTAL COST	$360	$295	$ 65

Source: JFCo Analysis

government influence with loss of freedom and imposition of red tape; invasion of community practice by outsiders; threats to status by the specter of employment in a hierarchy; and finally, possible reduction in earnings and standard of living. These are powerful deterrents which are being cited by alarmed physicians over the country.

While disadvantages cited are a real possibility, there is a consoling factor. If the overall system is economical, then everyone can gain by it—even the physicians. With a larger pie, everyone's piece can be bigger, and no one group needs to lose. It follows then that if the new sytem is an economic success, physicians stand to gain rather than lose.

The disadvantage of increased government influence is not one for the doctor alone; all society lives with that one. Industrial regulation is widespread, lamentable, more likely to grow in the future than to recede. If physicians have their earnings controlled, they can at least have the questionable satisfaction of knowing that businessmen or others will have their earnings controlled also. As for other interference, much will depend on how government agencies work with physicians. The right kind of cooperation could do wonders in cutting down red tape.

Change of practice could be a mixed blessing, and many doctors will welcome it. The opportunity to work in a group has advantages. Physicians can learn from each other, relieve one another of the otherwise continuous burden of caring for patients, and jointly acquire resources not otherwise affordable by single doctors. Size alone has advantages since it allows the group to organize so that each one can practice his specialty without unnecessary diversion, such as the solo practitioner diverted by bookkeeping problems when his nurse quits. Nor does the opportunity of working as a group necessarily mean the doctor must become a timecard-punching employee. As we mentioned earlier, there is more than one way to organize a practice, and the traditional organizational hierarchy need not be a part.

Placing more emphasis on preventive medicine should appeal to most doctors, not only for the good it can do, but for the dimension it adds to medical practice. Preventive practice will come as no stranger to the doctor; he already gives 20% or more of his time to it. What will be strange to some, and perhaps pleasant, is how prevention will be practiced. The routine tasks will be performed by paramedical personnel, leaving the physician more time for supervision and diagnosis. Automated monitoring, electronically controlled chemistry, computers and other devices will be used to extend the physicians' powers of surveillance and diagnosis. The job of educating patients will, in large part, be taken over by others so that the doctor can concentrate his limited time on the critical problems. Even the pesty job of shunting the hypochondriacs will be simplified by a modernized health surveillance system.

As for earnings, physicians apparently stand more to gain than lose in the new system. In spite of a popular misconception to the contrary, greater productivity generally results in greater earnings. Even with stringent government controls, it will be necessary to pay physicians what they are worth to attract a sufficient number into the industry. But most important, the government is already providing financial incentives to get doctors into group practice. As mentioned earlier, all states have recently passed professional service corporation acts which, along with federal legislation, give doctors and other professionals who incorporate unusual tax privileges. In *Medical Group News,* December 1971, Dale S. Carroll, JD, says, "A well designed pension or profit sharing plan can be flexible enough so that each doctor may invest as much or as little in each plan as he might desire. For example, either of two doctors earning $40,000 a year — or both of them — may contribute any amount or nothing up to $8,000 to the corporate pension or profit sharing plan according to the wishes of each." Dr. Carroll continues, "Incorporating will change no part of the clinic's operation, except that the physicians will vote through a board of directors."

To add to Dr. Carroll's statement, older doctors can set aside more than 20% of earnings, up to 100% in some cases, free of tax at the time of investment, and free of tax on any subsequent earnings or appreciation until the amounts are withdrawn after retirement. It doesn't take a financial genius to see the significance of the legislation.

Finally, physicians will find it easier to take on the establishment in groups. Through joint resources they will be able to hire counsel and other experts to represent them to the IRS man, the wage/price administrator, and patients who accuse them of malpractice. These and other advantages of group practice will be available in the scheme of things to come.

THE WELFARE OF OTHERS

Large corporations, hospitals, and others who undertake the general service functions in the system will get an opportunity to expand business, and if they go about it right, should find it respectable, pleasant, and profitable.

According to market studies, we should develop enough health maintenance centers (up to 10,000) for most of the population by 1985. We estimate that the general services required for an average center will be about $1.5 million yearly—making a total annual business of $15 billion in 1976 dollars. Entry capital into this business is relatively small, estimated at between 20% to 40% of annual revenues. Furthermore, the blueprint—even the HMO one—permits and encourages entrance of private capital in a configuration where a single corporation could be an asssociate service provider to many health centers by means of local service units.

The problem of creating and maintaining many service units is relatively simple because of replication features. Like the franchising business, one successful unit could be replicated many times. Finally, the new business is relatively safe, since health services will always be in demand; and government regulation will, at least, preclude ruinous competition.

Those who want to provide general services might find it profitable because of the following favorable factors:

1. A large market.
2. Low entry costs.
3. Private capital encouraged.

4. Profits allowed.
5. Units easily replicated.
6. Competition controlled.

Those who undertake the fiscal intermediary and insurance functions will find a market for their services of up to $10 billion in 1976
dollars annually; and those who take on both, the general services and
fiscal intermediary functions, will have a market that could be $25
billion annually. It is likely that companies now offering only medical
insurance will have a difficult time getting adjusted to the system.
Others like Kaiser and HIP will also have adjustments to make.
However, all companies now in the business are familiar with problems
they will encounter and should be able to successfully cope with them.
Once they have overcome the hurdles of change, they should find the
system rewarding.

TABLE 9-4
Potential Capital Requirements
For Group Practice
1976 — 1985
(Billions 1976 Dollars)

Planning	$ 2.0
Land and Buildings	8.0
Equipment	5.0
Working Capital	10.0
Start up Funds	2.0
Training and Other	3.0
TOTAL	$30.0

Source: JFCo Analysis

Not all of the amounts will come from new financing. Existing
facilities will be used and the government will furnish funds for planning, training, and some new facilities. The potential, however, for new
private capital is still large — about $20 billion.
    The $20 billion represents potential prime investment op-
portunities. According to the blueprint, rates of return should be high

enough to attract sufficient capital; facility loans will be eligible for 90% FHA guarantees; and much venture capital will be needed. Risk, even on venture capital, will be minimized by restrictions on competition planned. Also, another $20 billion or so will be required in the same period to modernize inpatient facilities.

To summarize, reward to private capitalists could be substantial for these reasons:

1. A large market.
2. High rates of return.
3. Capital gains opportunities.
4. Loan guarantees.
5. Competitive restrictions.

There are rewards for other providers: dentists, pharmacists, clinical labs, hospitals, and others. Demands for their services are likely to increase. Even hospitals faced with decreasing inpatient demands will have an opportunity to participate in the general service functions. Dentist and pharmacists can join centers as member providers and reap rewards similar to those of physicians. As preventive practice grows, clinical labs should enjoy a large increase in business.

Finally, there will be rewards for the sponsors of the new system: unions, companies, government agencies, schools, local communities, private practitioners, and others. They will have the satisfaction of spearheading the reconstruction of the medical industry.

REMOVING THE ROADBLOCKS

Since the incentives to rebuild the medical industry with CHOs are large, and the resources are abundant, it would seem that the job could be done rather quickly and it could, except for some serious roadblocks that must be cleared away.

Industry in general is somewhat paralyzed by the recent spate of government regulation over the medical industry, threats of regulation, anticipated programs such as upcoming NHI, and temporarily stalled programs such as HMO. Many of those who could contribute to the advancement of group practice, comprehensive care, and dual choice are simply waiting to see what is going to happen. The waiting time has already stretched out several years and it is conceivable that continued stalemate in Congress will stretch it out many more years.

Among those who are stalled are the physicians themselves, many of whom are also waiting to see what is going to happen. Whereas they might have gone ahead to form group practices in their own way, they have been detained by the imponderables in the picture. Futhermore, many have been turned off by misconceptions about group practice, spawned by HMO literature and the narrower prescriptions of some reformers and bureaucrats.

This handbook was designed to help remove some of these roadblocks: It shows how industry can go ahead without waiting for resolution of all government programs. The private sector can create health care centers that will do what HMOs can do, do it better, and, at the same time, satisfy physicians. It can make dual choice work by encouraging creation of centers that will give comprehensive care to the employees of industry for prepaid amounts paid through intermediaries or directly to centers at their option. Such a program would go a long way toward satisfying the objectives of reformers though not necessarily in the way they envision.

The handbook also shows physicians how to create practices that combine most of the advantages of solo practice with those of comprehensive group care. As an example, the following questions and answers were prepared to allay the fears of physicians contemplating such a group practice.

Questions and Answers of Physicians
Contemplating a CHO

Question: Do I have to give up any patients or assign them to a center I may join?

Answer: No.

Question: If I leave a center, can I take my patients with me?

Answer: Yes, if they want to leave also.

Question: Will I be an employee of the center?

Answer: No.

Question: Will my hours of work be regulated?

Answer: No.

Question: How will I get paid for my services?

Answer: The same as today. For services rendered to an enrollee in the plan, you will be paid by the center.

For those not in the plan, you will collect from the patient directly.

Question: Do I charge a fee for each service rendered?

Answer: Yes.

Question: Will my fees be regulated?

Answer: Only to the extent that fees are regulated under price controls.

Question: What if the patient is on capitation?

Answer: You charge a fee for each service the same as for others; but for patients on capitation, you will have to share surpluses or deficits in the capitation pool prorated in accordance with your share of pool payments.

Question: Do I have to accept capitation patients?

Answer: No.

Question: What are the advantages in capitation?

Answer: For Medicare and Medicaid groups capitation could insure payment of fees. For these groups and others, it could be an efficient way to practice, generating annual surpluses from which bonuses could be paid.

Question: Will insurance rates, particularly capitation rates, be adjustable?

Answer: Yes, subject to the same controls existing today.

Question: Who will my medical staff work for?

Answer: For you, and you will pay them.

Question: Can I join as a solo practitioner?

Answer: Yes, and if you are a partner, the partnership can join; and if a member of a corporation, the corporation can join. Joining the plan will not affect your present form of organization.

Question: Can I do my own booking, billing, and bookkeeping?

Answer: Yes. You can do all three if you want to, but you may find it economical to use the center's services for these chores.

Question: Must I move my office into the cneter?

Answer: Only if it is economical to do so.

Question: Must I buy the center's support services?

Answer: No. You will have an option to do so, and an obligation to give the center preference over outsiders for support services that it can economically provide.

Question: Can I get out of the center once I join?

Answer: Yes, subject to contract terms which specify reasonable advance notification.

Question: Do I have to invest in the center?

Answer: Not unless you want to.

Question: What do I do with my present lease?

Answer: The plan provides a reasonable funding pool for terminating leases.

Question: Can I retain my hospital staff appointments?

Answer: Yes.

In short, the handbook was written as a guide to development of group practice in the next decade. It should help overcome some of the fears, uncertainties, and other roadblocks to the emerging system of medical care.

Appendix A
Planning Tables

ABOUT THE TABLES

The following set of tables is useful in planning the development of health care enterprises. Together with census data of a neighborhood and other information about local health care resources, they can be used to generate useful data on a given market and on a range of feasible health care center configurations to serve the market.

As illustrated in the case example of Appendix B, the tables can be used to virtually generate a complete advanced plan for a health care enterprise from readily ascertainable information about a neighborhood. While it takes some skill to use the tables in planning—a skill possesed by most experienced planners—the tables have been used in a semi-automated planning generator that turns out a completed document in a few hours' time from information gathered on a questionnaire.

The inexperienced planner should be warned, however, that canned plans worked out from tables can be misleading. No matter how refined, planning factors are based on averages that may not all pertain to a given situation. The averages also change from year to year, especially costing factors, which can vary in some cases 100% or more. Finally, every table is built on assumptions that don't always apply to the case at hand.

Still the planning tables and canned planning are extremely useful to the skilled planner. They give him a quick grasp of the overall parameters of a problem, a useful check on final results, and last, but not least, a convenient way to fill in some of the gaps.

For those not familiar with planning, this last point may come as a surprise. Filling in the gaps with canned data would appear to be risky; and it is to a certain extent. But as every skilled planner knows, all the information needed to construct a plan is seldom, if ever, available.

The alternative to "dying on the job" is to fill in the gaps as well as possible with prudent estimates. And the tables are a big help in this regard.

Finally, the tables provide an excellent checklist in the planning process—indicating not only the steps that have to be followed in the planning process but alternative goals that might be selected as a plan is generated.

TABLE 1
Disorder Prevalence
By Age Group as Ratios of Age Group Population

Item	0-20	21-30	31-40	41-50	51-65	Over 65
Population--% of Total	37	17	14	11	11	10
Obesity	.15	.20	.30	.40	.40	.20
Anxiety, Tension, Depression	.05	.10	.15	.15	.15	.10
Muscle, Joint, Bone Disorder	.03	.05	.10	.15	.30	.40
Cardiovascular Disorder	.02	.04	.06	.10	.20	.40
Hypertension (1)	.02	.07	.16	.36	.50	.40
Alcoholism	.005	.05	.06	.08	.10	.08
Diabetes	.02	.03	.04	.06	.08	.08
Blood Disorder (Other)	.02	.04	.04	.04	.04	.04
Psychiatric Disorder (Other)	.01	.02	.03	.03	.03	.04
Urological Disorder	.005	.02	.02	.03	.05	.10
Liver Disorder	.005	.01	.02	.04	.06	.06
Pulmonary Disorder (3)	.01	.01	.01	.015	.02	.02
Other Long Term Disorder (4)	.03	.09	.09	.085	.10	.15
Total	.375	.73	1.08	1.54	2.03	2.07
Acute Illnesses	.047	.030	.020	.020	.018	.015
Accident Recuperation	.009	.006	.005	.005	.005	.005
Pregancy	.006	.035	.012	—	—	—
Infant Illnesses (2)	.003	—	—	—	—	—
Total	.065	.071	.037	.025	.023	.020

Notes: (1) All Cases—Divide by 2 for severe cases.
(2) Under one year.
(3) Includes tuberculosis, emphysema, neoplasm.
(4) Includes asthma, bronchitis and others except hearing and vision cases.

TABLE 2
Disorder Prevalence
By Age Group as Ratios of Total Population

Disorder	Age Class							
	0-20	21-30	31-40	41-50	51-65	Over 65	Total	18-65
Population-%	37	17	14	11	11	10	100	58
Obesity	.055	.034	.042	.044	.044	.020	.239	.170
Tension, Anxiety, Depression	.018	.017	.021	.017	.017	.010	.100	.088
Muscle, Joint, Bone Disorder	.011	.009	.014	.017	.033	.040	.124	.075
Cardiovascular Disorder	.007	.007	.008	.011	.022	.040	.095	.049
Hypertension (acute)	.004	.006	.011	.020	.028	.020	.089	.066
Alcoholism	.002	.008	.008	.009	.011	.008	.046	.037
Diabetes	.007	.005	.006	.007	.009	.008	.042	.028
Blood Disorder	.007	.007	.006	.004	.004	.004	.032	.022
Psychiatric Disorder	.004	.003	.003	.003	.003	.004	0.20	.013
Urological Disorder	.002	.003	.003	.003	.006	.010	.027	.015
Liver Disorder	.002	.002	.003	.004	.007	.006	.024	.016
Pulmonary Disorder	.004	.002	.001	.002	.002	.002	.013	.008
Other Long Term Disorder (1)	.011	.015	.012	.010	.011	.015	.074	.051
Total Long Term	.134	.118	.138	.151	.197	.187	.925	.638
Acute Illness	.018	.005	.003	.002	.002	.002	.032	.014
Accident Recuperation	.003	.001	.001	.001	.001	.001	.008	.005
Pregnancy	.002	.006	.002	---	---	---	.010	.010
Infant Illnesses (2)	.001	—	—	---	-	—	.001	---
Total Short Term	.024	.012	.006	.003	.003	.003	.051	.029
Total Illness	.158	.130	.144	.154	.200	.190	.976	.677

Notes: (1) Does not include hearing and vision defects amounting to 7.2% to 4.7%, respectively, for the entire population.

(2) Under one year.

TABLE 3
Care Administered, Yearly Rates

ITEM	FORMULA		UNITS	UNIT COST
Deliveries	Per Pregnant Patient		1.33	$ 600.00
Major Surgery	Per 1000 Age 0-20		10	$1000.00
	Patients 21-65		25	
	over 65		40	
Minor Surgery	Per 1000 Patients		60	$ 250.00
Physician Office and House Visits	Per Patient Listed for Well-Care		0.2	
	Per Chronically Ill Patient		1.5	$ 15.00
	Per Acutely Ill Patient		60.0(2)	
	Per Accident Patient		60.0(2)	
	Per Pregnant Patient		16.0	
Physician Hospital Visits	Per Bed		400.0	$ 15.00
Dental Visits	Per Patient Listed		2.0	$ 20.00
Prescription Drugs (1)	Per Patient Listed		6.0	$ 6.00
Clinical Tests (1)	Per Patient Listed		10	$ 1.50
X-rays (excl. dental) (1)	Per Patient Listed		0.6	$ 20.00
Short Term Hospital Days	Per Patient Age 0-20		0.5	$ 160.00
	21-65		1.3	
	65 & over		4.0	
Care Facility Days	Percent of Hospital Days		80%	$ 40.00
Prophylactics and Medical Supplies (1)	Per Patient Listed		—	$ 3.00
Psychotherapy	Per Patient Listed		—	$ 8.00
Physical Therapy (1)	Per Patient Listed		—	$ 10.00
Related Fiscal Services	Percent of Total Cost		—	4%

Notes:

(1)   Excludes hospital furnished items.

(2)   Amounts to 1.15 calls per week converted to an annual basis.

TABLE 4
Adjustments to Care Administered
for Patient Groups

GROUPS	ADJUSTMENT TO TABLES 1 THRU 3
Middle Income and Affluent Whites	0.9 x Table Values
Low Income and Blacks (1)	1.5 x Table Values

Note:

(1)   For those currently on public programs only. Varies considerably from state to state.

TABLE 5
Disease Costs ($ Billions Annually)

DISORDER	CARE	MORTALITY	ABSENTEE-ISM	INEFFI-CIENCY	TOTAL
		COST OF DISORDER			
Obesity	0.5	—	—	6.0	6.5
Tension, Anxiety & Depression	1.5	2.5	3.0	7.0	4.0
Muscle, Joints & Bone Disorders	4.0	2.0	3.0	6.0	15.0
Cardiovascular Disorder	8.0	27.0	4.0	9.0	48.0
Hypertension (acute)	2.0	—	2.5	5.0	9.5
Alcoholism	2.0	2.0	7.0	10.0	21.0
Diabetes	3.0	3.0	1.0	1.0	8.0
Blood Disorder	1.7	0.7	0.7	1.5	4.6
Psychiatric Disorder	4.0	0.8	15.0	1.0	20.8
Urological Disorder	2.6	1.0	0.4	1.0	5.0
Liver Disorder	1.7	0.7	0.5	0.5	3.4
Pulmonary Disorder	3.3	1.0	0.2	0.2	4.7
Drug Addiction	2.0	5.0	3.0	2.0	12.0
Venereal Disease	0.7	1.5	0.7	0.7	3.6
Cancer	9.0	8.5	0.8	0.8	19.1
Stroke	2.7	2.0	0.2	0.3	5.2
Other Long Term Disorders	11.3	4.3	1.0	2.5	19.1
Preventive Care and Other*	40.0	—	—	—	40.0
Acute Illness	15.0	10.0	30.0	1.0	56.0
Accidents & Violence	10.0	12.0	9.0	1.0	32.0
Pregnancy	5.0	1.0	3.0	3.5	12.5
Grand Total	130.0	85.0	85.0	60.0	360.0

Note:

*Preventive Care, $10.00; Dental Care, $8.00; Prosthetics, $3.00; Fiscal Services, $5.00; Public Health Services, $5.00; Research, $3.00; Net Capital Expansion, $3.00; Education, $1.00; Other, $2.00.

TABLE 6
Improvement Goals in 10 Years
Reduction in Prevalence of Illness

Item	% Improvement
Obesity	50
Nervous Tension	33
Muscles, Joints, Bones	33
Heart	25
Hypertension	25
Alcoholism (Active)	50
Diabetes	-
Other Blood Disorder	10
Psychiatric Disorder	20
Urological Disorder	33
Liver Disorder	25
Pulmonary Disorder	50
Drug Addiction (Active)	50
Venereal Disease	50
Other Long Term Disorder	33
Acute Illness	33
Accidents	10
Pregnancy Cases	20
Infant Illnesses (under 1 year)	20

TABLE 7
Improvement Goals in 10 Years
Change in Care Administered

Item	% Change
Deliveries	-20%
Major Surgery	-25%
Minor Surgery	-33%
Physician Visits	-25%
Dental Visits	-
Prescription Drugs	20%
Clinical Tests	+100%
X-Ray	+33%
Short Term Hospital Days	-33%
Extended Care	+50%
Prosthetics & Medical Supplies	-
Psychotherapy	-
Physical Therapy	-33%
Patient Education	+ ($5 per person yearly)
Environmental Protection	+ ($3 per person yearly)
Related Fiscal Services	-(100)%

TABLE 8
Improvement Goals in 10 Years
Health Related Costs

Item	% Improvement
Premature Mortality Cost	33
Absenteeism Cost	25
Occupational Inefficiency Cost	25

TABLE 9
Health Care Organization Services
All Services

1. Medical Services
   Primary Care
      General
      Adult Care
      Baby Care
      Dental Care
      Eye Care
   Specialty Care
      In Patient
      Surgery
      Therapy
2. Drug Distribution
3. Medical Education
   Patients
   Providers

4. Health Surveillance
   Periodic Examinations
   Special Examinations
   Diagnostic Analyses
   Medical History
5. Chemical Lab Services
6. X-Ray Lab Services
7. Transportation Services
   Patients (Ambulance & Other)
   Providers & Employees
   Materials

8. Facility Services
   Accomodation
   Custody
   Maintenance
   Cleaning
   Groundskeeping
   Repairs
   Supply Services
   Utilities
   Building Operations
9. Insurance Services
   Marketing
   Claims Services
   Collections &
      Distributions
   Risk Services
   Other Services

10. Administrative Services
   Direction
   Engineering & Planning
   Control Services
      Service Control
      Quality Control
      Cost Control
      Utilization Control
   Purchasing Services
   Employee Services
      Recruitment
      Employment
      Training
      Employee Health Services
      Estate Building Services
      Recreation
      Food & Beverage Services
      Other Benefits
   Communication Services
      Reception Services
      Switchboard Services
      Teledata Services
      Paging Services
      Mail Services
      Messenger Services
   Public Relations Services
   Legal Services

   Accounting Services
      Budgeting
      Billing & Credit
      Payroll
      Payables
      Cashiering
      Cost Accounting
      Bookkeeping
      Reporting
      Auditing
      Insurance Services
      Tax Services
   Library Services
   Data Processing Services
      Diagnostic Analyses
      Procedure Look Up
      Prescription Look Up
      Patient History
      Remote Booking
      Scheduling
      Billing
      Bookkeeping
      Management Reports
      Listings
      Technical Data

TABLE 10
Health Care Organization Service
Office Practice Only

1. MAIN SERVICES:

Provided Inhouse	Provided Inhouse or Outside	Provided Outside Only
Primary Care (O&O)	Dental Care	
Preventive	Dental Care	
Curative	Dental Care	
Arrestive	Dental Care	
Rehabilitative	Dental Care	
Specialty Care (O&O)		
		Major Surgery
Minor Surgery (L)	In Patient Care (L)	Minor Surgery (R)
	Physical Therapy (L)	Inpatient Care (R)
	Psycho therapy (L)	Physical Therapy (R)
	Other Care (L)	Psychotherapy (R)
Drug Distribution (L)		Other Care (R)
Medical Education		Drug Distribution (R)

2. SUPPORT SERVICES:

Provided Inhouse	Provided Inhouse or Outside	Provided Outside Only
Health Surveillance		
Chem Lab Service (L)		Chem Lab Service (R)
X-Ray Lab Diagnostic (L)		X-Ray Lab (R)
	Facility Services (L)	Facility Services (R)
	Transportation	Transportation
	Services (L)	Services (R)
Fiscal Services (L)		Fiscal Services (R)
Administrative		Administrative
Services (L)		Services (R)

Notes: O&O — Office & Outpatient Care, including emergency care
   L   — Limited service only
   R   — Remainder of services partially performed inhouse

TABLE 11
Health Care Organization Units

---

1. Health Plan Unit

2. Medical Unit
   Primary Care Offices
   Specialty Care Offices
   Dental Offices
   Therapy Offices

3. Service Unit
   Executive
   Education
   Outpatient Ward
   Patient Examination Ward
   Chem Lab
   X-Ray Lab
   Drug
   Building Services
      Custody
      Transportation
      Supply
      Maintenance
   Administrative Services
      Administrative Control
      Communications
      Record Keeping
      Data Processing

4. Fiscal Unit
   Management Office
   Sales
   Claims & Remittances
   Insurance

5. Capital Unit

6. Consulting Unit

TABLE 12
Health Care Organization Contracts

---

1. Organization Charter

2. Professional Licenses

3. Certificate-of-Need

4. Building Permits

5. Enrollee Contracts:
   > General Public
   > Medicare
   > Medicaid

6. Provider Contracts:
   > Professional Providers—Plan
   > Professional Providers—Non-Plan
   > Fiscal Unit
   > Capital Unit
   > Service Unit
   > Consulting Unit
   > Suppliers

7. Employee Contracts

8. Other Contracts:
   > Insurance—Catastrophe
   > Insurance—Liability
   > Insurance—Fire & Theft
   > Insurance—Life
   > Estate & Retirement Plans

TABLE 13
Health Care Organization Functions

ESTABLISHMENT UNIT	MUST BE PERFORMED IN UNIT	MAY BE PERFORMED IN UNIT OR ELSEWHERE

Health Plan Unit	Policy Making
	Execution of Plan Contracts
	  Providers
	  Enrollees
	Provision of Care for Enrollees
	Acquisition of Care from
	        Providers
	Collection for Services
	        Provided
	Remittance for Services
	        Acquired
	Performance Evaluation	

Medical Unit	Planning of the Unit
	Direction of the Unit
	Control of the Unit:
	  Scheduling Operations
	  Booking Patients (L)
	  Quality Control (L)
	  Cost Control
	  Utilization Control
	  Performance Evaluation (L)
	Medical History (L)
	Patient Examination:
	  Special (L)
	  Preventive (L)
	Diagnosis (L)
	Consultation of Patients
	Prescription
	Prognosis
	References (L)
	Treatment (L)
	
	Communications (L)
		Control:
		
		  Booking Patients (R)
		
		Patient Examination:
		  Special (R)
		
		Diagnosis (R)
		
		References (R)
		Treatment (R)
		Minor Surgery (L)
		Therapy (L)
		Outpatient Aid (L)
		Transportation
		Communications (R)

Notes:
  L—Limited Execution
  R—Remainder of Execution

TABLE 13
Health Care Organization Functions (Continued)

ESTABLISHMENT UNIT	MUST BE PERFORMED IN UNIT	MAY BE PERFORMED IN UNIT OR ELSEWHERE

Medical Unit (continued)	Personnel Functions (L)
	Purchasing (L)
	Supply (L)
	Accounting (L)
	Financial (L)
	Legal (L)
	Medical Info Processing:
	  Patient History (L)
	  Technical Data (L)
	Education—Medical
	  Patients (L)
	  Practitioners (L)
	  Employees (L)
		Personnel Functions (R)
		Purchasing (R)
		Supply (R)
		Accounting (R)
		Financial (R)
		Legal (R)
		Medical Info Processing:
		  Patient History (R)
		  Technical Data (R)
		Education—Medical
		
		  Practitioners (R)
		  Employees (R)

Service Unit	Planning
	  Overall Operation
	  Service Unit Only
	Direction of Unit
	Control:
	  Scheduling Operations—
	  Overall
	  Service Unit Only
	
	  Quality Control—
	  Overall
	  Service Unit Only
	  Cost Control—
	  Overall
	  Service Unit Only
	  Utilization—
	  Overall
	  Service Unit Only
	  Performance Evaluation—
	  Overall
	  Service Unit Only
		Control:
		
		Booking Patients (L)
		
		Outpatient Functions:
		  Patient Examination
		  Diagnosis
		  Consultation
		  Prescription
		  Referrals
		  Treatment
		  Emergency Aid

TABLE 13
Health Care Organization Functions (Continued)

ESTABLISHMENT UNIT	MUST BE PERFORMED IN UNIT	MAY BE PERFORMED IN UNIT OR ELSEWHERE
Service Unit (continued)		Health Surveillance: Medical History (L) Patient Examination (L)
	Laboratory Testing Diagnostic X-Ray Drug Distribution Education: Patients (L)	
		Practitioners Employees
	Transportation Patients (L) Providers & Employees (L) Materials (L)	Transportation
	Communications: Reception (L) Telephone (L) Teledata (L) Paging (L) Mail (L) Messenger (L)	Communications: Reception (R)
	Personnel Functions:	Personnel Functions: Employment (L) Training (L)
	Health Care Recreation Estate Building Food & Beverage Other Benefits	
	Purchasing (L)	Purchasing (R)
	Building Service Functions: Operation Maintenance: Cleaning Groundskeeping Repairs Supply Services (L) Building Operations	

TABLE 13
Health Care Organization Functions (Continued)

ESTABLISHMENT UNIT	MUST BE PERFORMED IN UNIT	MAY BE PERFORMED IN UNIT OR ELSEWHERE
Service Unit (continued)	Accounting:	Accounting:
	Budgeting—	Budgeting—
	Overall	
	Service Unit Only	Of Other Units (L)
	Billing & Credit (L)	Billing & Credit (R)
	Payroll (L)	Payroll (R)
	Payables (L)	Payables (R)
	Cashiering (L)	Cashiering (R)
	Cost Accounting (L)	Cost Accounting (R)
	Bookkeeping (L)	Bookkeeping (R)
	Reporting—	Reporting—
	Overall	
	Service Unit Only	On Other Units
	Auditing	
	Insurance	
	Tax Services	
	Public Relations	
	Legal Functions	
		Technical Info Processing:
		Diagnosis (L)
		Prescription (L)
		Referrals (L)
		Patient History (L)
	Data Processing Functions:	Data Processing:
		Diagnostic Analysis (L) (R)
		Procedure Look Up (L) (R)
		Prescription Look Up (L) (R)
		Patient History (L) (R)
	Booking (L)	Booking (R)
	Scheduling (L)	Scheduling (R)
	Billing (L)	Billing (R)
	Bookkeeping (L)	Bookkeeping (R)
	Management Reports (L)	Management Reports (R)
	Listings (L)	Listings (R)

TABLE 13
Health Care Organization Functions (Continued)

ESTABLISHMENT UNIT	MUST BE PERFORMED IN UNIT	MAY BE PERFORMED IN UNIT OR ELSEWHERE
Fiscal Unit	Patient Enrollment Marketing (L) Claims Collections & Distributions Insurance—Catastrophic Insurance—Stop Loss	

TABLE 14
Health Care Organization Systems

---

1. Control Systems:
    Policy Formulation
    Operational Planning
    Financial Planning
    Scheduling Systems
        Family Health Management
        Patient Booking
        Referral Systems
    Quality Control
    Cost Control
    Performance Evaluation
    Management Reporting Systems
    Auditing Systems

2. Service Systems:
    Primary Care Systems
    Specialty Care Systems
    Outpatient Systems—Regular
    Outpatient Systems—Emergency
    Patient Examination Systems
    Laboratory Systems—Chemical
    Laboratory Systems—X-Ray

3. People Systems:
    Enrollment Systems
    Inpatient Systems
    Physical Therapy Systems
    Psychotherapy Systems
    Recruitment Systems
    Employment Systems
    Training Systems

4. Goods & Materials Systems:
    Medical Supplies
    Office Supplies
    Building Supplies
    Drug Distribution
    Food & Beverage

5. Transportation Systems:
    Patient Transportation
    Employee Transportation
    Supplies Transportation
    Parking Lot

6. Plant, Equipment & Grounds:
    Custody Systems
    Power & Light
    Water
    Gas
    Heat
    Air Conditioning
    Disposal
    Maintenance
    Construction, Alteration
        & Demolition

7. Money & Credit Systems:
    Billing & Claims
    Receipts & Disbursements
    Insurance
    Compensation
    Estate & Retirement

TABLE 14
Health Care Organizations Systems (Continued)

---

8. Information Systems:
   Technical Information Storage
   & Retrieval—
   Rules & Regulations
   Procedures—Medical
   Procedures—Other
   Pharmacopoeia
   Supply Catalogs
   Listings—
      Codes
      Fees & Prices
      Rates & Costs
      Standards
      Specifications
      Patient Lists
      Employee Lists
      Supplier Lists
      Investor Lists
      Telephone Lists
   Clippings
   Magazines & Books
   Planning Systems—
      Establishment Plans
      Organization Plans
      System Plans
      Procedures & Programs
      Building Plans
      Contract Plans
         Medical Service
         Provider Contracts
         Employee Contracts
   Patient History Systems
   Education Systems—
      Patients
      Providers
   General Correspondence

9. Data Processing Systems:
   Diagnostic Analysis
   Procedure Look Up
   Prescription Look Up
   Patient History
   Scheduling
   Booking
   Billing
   Bookkeeping
   Management Reports
   Listings

10. Communications Systems:
   Reception System
   Telephone System
   Paging System
   Teledata System
   Mail System
   Messenger System

TABLE 15
Health Care Organization Manpower

MANPOWER CLASSIFICATION	QUANTITY PER PRACTITIONER (P) PER % ENROLLED					
	8 Ps		16 Ps		24 Ps	
	25%	100%	25%	100%	25%	100%
Office Care						
Primary Care Physicians	4	4	8	8	12	12
Other Physicians	2	2	4	4	6	6
Dentists	2	2	4	4	6	6
Head Nurses	8	8	16	16	24	24
Asst. Nurses	4	4	8	8	12	12
Outpatient Care						
Asst. Doctors	1/2	1/2	1/2	1	1/2	1 1/2
Head Nurses	1/2	1/2	1/2	1	1	1 1/2
Medical Support						
Pharmacists	1	2	2	4	3	6
Laboratory Technicians	1	1	2	2	3	3
Radiology Technicians	1	1	2	2	3	3
Asst. Doctors	1/2	1/2	1/2	1	1/2	1 1/2
Head Nurses	1/2	1/2	1/2	1	1	1 1/2
Educators	-	1	-	2	1	2
Building Services						
Custodians	1	1	1	1	1	1
Drivers	1	1	2	2	2	2
Others	-	-	1	1	2	2
Administration						
Administrator	1	1	1	1	1	1
Admin. Asst.	-	-	-	1	1	2
Bkkpr./Clerk/Secy.	2	4	2	6	3	9
Receptionist/Switchboard	-	1	1	2	1	2
GRAND TOTAL	30	35	56	68	84	99

Notes:　The table is based on a comprehensive care center with the
following specifications:
1. Office practice only
2. Dental and drug coverage is optional
3. One-half of the specialty care range only is
covered inhouse

TABLE 16
Health Care Organization Equipment
Minimum Requirements
$000

| ITEM | 8 Practitioners | | |
| | Fixed | Mobile | |
		Deployed	Central
Office Practice		90	25
Outpatient Ward			10
Pharmacy			5
Education			5
Screening Lab			15
Lab-X-Ray			15
Lab-Chemical			10
Transportation			5
Communications			5
Heating & Air Conditioning	20		
Power & Light	30		
Business Equipment			10
Total	50	90	105

TABLE 16
Health Care Organization Equipment
Minimum Requirements
$000 (Continued)

	16 Practitioners			24 Practitioners	
Fixed	Mobile		Fixed	Mobile	
	Deployed	Central		Deployed	Central
	180	50		270	80
		15			20
		10			15
		10			15
		20			25
		25			35
		15			20
		10			15
		10			15
30			40		
45			60		
		15			20
75	180	180	100	270	260

TABLE 17
Health Care Organization Space

100% Utilization

Item	Unit	Space Per Practitioner (P)				
		8 Ps	16 Ps	24 Ps	48 Ps	96 Ps
Office Care Center						
Office Practice	000 Sq Ft	5.6	11.2	16.8	33	66
Outpatients	,,	0.8	1.6	2.4	5	5
Education	,,	.2	.4	.4	1	1
Screening Lab	,,	.7	1.4	2.0	3	4
Pharmacy	,,	.4	.4	.4	1	2
Lab X-Ray	,,	.4	.4	.4	1	2
Lab Chemical	,,	.4	.4	.4	1	2
Reception	,,	.4	.4	.4	1	2
Accounting	,,	.4	.5	.6	1	1
EDP	,,	-	-	.4	1	1
Plant Services	,,	.4	.4	.4	1	2
Executive Staff	,,	.3	.4	.6	1	1
Sub-Total		10.0	17.5	25.2	50	89
Hospital	,,	20.0	32.0	46.0	94	170
Extended Care Facility	,,	5.0	8.0	11.0	23	40
Total—Bldg. Space	,,	35.0	57.5	82.0	167	299
Office Care Center	Acres	1	2	3	6	9
Hospital	,,	2	4	6	12	20
Extended Care Facility	,,	1	1	2	3	5
Total—Land	,,	4	7	11	21	34

Note: The table is based on the equivalent of one full-time-equivalent primary care physician for each non-primary care practitioner employed. Also it assumes 1800 patients per primary care physician or 900 patients per practitioner.

TABLE 18
Supplies

---

1. Medical Supplies
    Outside Services
        Surgical Supplies
        Drugs
        Biologics
    Diagnostic Kits
    Linens & Uniforms
    Other

2. Laboratory Supplies
    Outside Services
    Glassware
    Reagents
    Test Kits
    X-Ray Film
    Uniforms
    Other

3. Pharmacy Supplies
    Drugs
    Capsules
    Containers
    Labels
    Packaging
    Forms
    Other

4. Building Supplies
    Utilities
        Gas
        Electricity
        Other
    Maintenance Materials
        Outside Services
        Tools and Implements
        Building Materials
        Replacement Parts
        Cleaning Supplies
        Other

Transportation Supplies
    Outside Services
    Tools and Implements
    Gasoline and Oil
    Spare Parts
    Other
Material Handling Supplies
    Tools and Implements
    Packing Materials
    Other
Food and Beverage
Other

5. Office Supplies
    Outside Services
    Telephone
    Postage
    Stationery
    Tapes and Cassettes

6. Informational Supplies
    Library Materials
        Books
        Journals & Magazines
        Trade Papers
        Other
    Educational Materials
        Courses
        Displays
        Other

7. Financial & Other Supplies
    Insurance
    Other Benefits
    Consulting
    Licenses & Dues
    Travel
    Other

TABLE 19
Health Care Organization Preliminary Planning Events

EVENT	BEGIN	END	RESPON-SIBILITY	CONSULTING MANWEEKS	OUTSIDE COST $K
Explore Proposition	1	4	P	—	—
Set Up Organization	5	10	C	1	1.5
Set Up Organization	—	—	L	.5	1.0
Make Feasibility Survey	6	7	C	2	3.0
Prepare Preliminary Plan	3	9	C	4	6.0
Get Approval of Plan	10	11	C	1	1.5
File Plan (1)	12	13	C	1	1.0
Apply for Planning Grant (1)	12	13	C	1	1.5
Slack Time for Approval	14	26	—	—	—
Total	1	26	—	10.5	$15.5

Notes:

(1)   For government grant only.
C—Consultants
L—Lawyers
P—Principals

TABLE 20
Health Care Organization Advanced Planning Events

EVENT	WEEK BEGIN	END	RESPON-SIBILITY	CONSULTING MANWEEKS	OUTSIDE COST $K
Make Market Survey	1	2	C	4	6
Prepare Advanced Plan	3	5	C	6	9
Get Approval of Principals	6	6	C	.6	1
File Development Plan with State	6	7	C	.3	.5
Apply for Certificate-of–Need	6	7	C	.3	.5
Investigate Sources of Funding	6	9	C	2	3
Draw up Financial Documents	10	12	L	3	6
Apply for Development Funding	13	14	P	—	—
Slack Time for Funding	15	26	—	—	—
Total	1	26	—	15.2	$25K

Notes:
    C—Consultants
    L—Lawyers
    P—Principals

TABLE 21
Health Care Organization Implementation Events
Pre Start-Up Phase

EVENT	WEEK BEGIN	END	RESPON-SIBILITY	CONSULTING MANWEEKS	OUTSIDE COST $K
Realign Organization	1	6	C	2	3.0
Realign Organization			L	3	6.0
Realign Organization			P	—	
Recruit Key Staff	1	8	C	4	6.0
Recruit Key Staff			P	—	—
Recruit Key Staff			A	—	—
Get Temporary Space	1	8	A	—	—
Contract with Providers	1	12	L	2	4.0
Contract with Providers			C	4	6.0
Contract with Providers			A	—	—
Establish Line of Credit	1	12	C	2	3.0
Establish Line of Credit			A	—	—
Design Systems	1	26	C	26	39.0
Design Systems			A	—	—
Create Legal Documentation	6	26	L	6	12.0
Contract with Intermediary	13	20	L	2	4.0
Contract with Intermediary			C	2	3.0
Contract with Intermediary			A	—	—
Detail Organization	16	26	C	4	6.0
Detail Organization			A	—	—
Recruit Subscribers	16	26	C	2	3.0
Recruit Subscribers			A	—	—
Negotiate Group Subscrip.	16	26	L	2	4.0
Negotiate Group Subscrip.			C	2	3.0
Negotiate Group Subscrip.			A	—	—
Pre-Design Facilities	16	26	C	4	6.0
Pre-Design Facilities			E	15	20.0
Pre-Design Facilities			A	—	—
Negotiate Construction	22	26	A	—	—
Apply to FHA (1)	22	26	C	2	3.0
Apply to FHA (1)			A	—	—
Prepare Financial Plan	22	26	C	4	6.0
Total				88	$137

Notes:
  (1)   if needed
  L—Lawyers
  C—Consultants
  A—Administrative Staff
  E—Engineers

TABLE 22
Health Care Organization Implementation Events
Post Start-Up Phase

EVENT	WEEK BEGIN	END	RESPON-SIBILITY	CONSULTING MANWEEKS	OUTSIDE COST $K
8PPs					
Start-Up	1	52	A	—	—
Install Systems	1	36	C	8	$12
Install Systems			A	—	—
Recruit Initial Staff	1	36	C	4	6
Recruit Initial Staff			A	—	—
Train Initial Staff	1	36	C	4	6
Train Initial Staff			A	—	—
Construction-Phase I	1	36	B	—	—
Shake Down	52	104	C	8	12
Shake Down			A	—	—
Total				24	$36
16PPs					
Start-Up	1	52	A	—	—
Install Systems	1	36	C	12	18
Install Systems			A	—	—
Recruit Initial Staff	1	36	C	6	9
Recruit Initial Staff			A	—	—
Train Initial Staff	1	36	C	6	9
Train Initial Staff			A	—	—
Construction-Phase I	1	36	B	—	—
Construction-Phase II	36	62	B	—	—
Shake Down	36	104	C	12	18
Total				36	$54
24PPs					
Start-Up	1	52	A	—	—
Install Systems	0	36	C	16	24
Install Systems			A	—	—
Recruit Initial Staff	0	36	C	8	12
Recruit Initial Staff			A	—	—
Train Initial Staff	0	36	C	8	12
Train Initial Staff			A	—	—
Construction-Phase I	0	36	B	—	—
Construction-Phase II	36	62	B	—	—
Construction-Phase III	62	88	B	—	—
Shake Down	36	104	C	16	24
Total				48	$72

Notes: C—Consultants
        B—Builders
        A—Administrator

TABLE 23
Health Care Organization Patients by Practice
Characteristics
000s Patients

PRIMARY CARE PRACTITIONERS (1)	TOTAL PRACTITIONERS	NUMBER OF PATIENTS 000s	
		Medically Needy (2)	Others
8	8-24	4000	8000
16	16-48	8000	16000
24	24-72	12000	24000
32	32-96	16000	32000

Notes:

(1)   Full-time-equivalency which includes the part-time services of specialists doing primary care work. Also includes the services of parameds doing primary care work.

(2)   Blacks and hispanics in general, Medicaid and medically indigent, and elderly patients.

TABLE 24
Health Care Organization Revenue Factors

ITEM	PERIOD	YEARLY INCIDENCE AND $ RATES	
Outpatient Visits	All Periods	1.00/Enrollee .33/Non-enrollee	@$15 ea. to Service Unit @$ 5 ea. to Medical Unit
Periodic Physicals	At Start	.40/Enrollee .13/Non-enrollee	@$50 ea. to Service Unit
	Later On	.50/Enrollee .17/Non-enrollee	@$50 ea. to Service Unit
Drug Purchases	All Periods	3.00/Enrollee 1.00/Non-enrollee	@$ 6 ea. to Service Unit
Stat Lab Tests	All Periods	1.00/Enrollee .30/Non-enrollee	@$ 5 ea. to Service Unit
Diagnostic X-Rays	All Periods	1.00/Enrollee 0.3 /Non-enrollee	@$10 ea. to Service Unit
Enrollee Payments	At Start	$480/Enrollee Year to Plan Unit $100/Enrollee Year to Medical Unit $260/Enrollee Year to Other Providers	
	Later on	$240/Enrollee Year to Other Providers	
Fee-For-Service Payments	All Periods	$100/Non-enrollee + $20/Patient to Medical Unit	
Insurance Income	All	5% of Capitation Rate to Fiscal Unit	
Rentals-Space -Equip.	All Periods	$10/square foot per year to Plan Unit $ 5/square foot per year to Plan Unit	
Administrative Services	All Periods	2% of Revenues to Service Unit	

Notes: For a comprehensive care clinic with the following characteristics:

1. Does not cover long term care in an institution.
2. 25% of the patients enrolled at the start;
   87.5% of the patients enrolled later on.
3. 20% medically needy patients involved.
4. Drug and dental coverage is optional. One half subscribe to each.
5. All enrollee income paid to the Plan Unit and redistributed.

TABLE 25
Health Care Organization Cumulative Requirements by Quarter

ITEM	MEASURE	PRELIMINARY PLANNING		ADVANCED PLANNING	
		1	2	3	4
ALL UNITS					
Enrollees	Units	—	—	—	—
Other Patients	Units	—	—	—	—
Total	Units	—	—	—	—
HMO					
Adm. Director	Units	—	—	—	1/4
Clerk Secretary	Units	—	—	—	1/4
Rented Space	(000 sq ft)	—	—	—	4.4
Building (2)	$000	—	—	—	—
Equipment (2)	$000	—	—	—	—
Systems (2)	$000	15	25	270	345
SERVICE UNIT					
Administrator	Units	—	—	—	3/4
Clerk Secretary	Units	—	—	—	3/4
Adm. Assistants	Units	—	—	—	—
Educators	Units	—	—	—	—
Asst. Doctors	Units	—	—	—	—
Head Nurses	Units	—	—	—	—
Pharmacists	Units	—	—	—	1
Lab Technicians	Units	—	—	—	1
Radiology Tech.	Units	—	—	—	—
Bldg. Support Prsnl.	Units	—	—	—	—
Admin. Support Prsnl.	Units	—	—	—	—
Rented Space	(000 sq. ft)	—	—	—	4.4
Capital (2)	$000	—	—	—	250
MEDICAL UNIT					
Practitioners	Units	—	—	—	—
Head Nurses	Units	—	—	—	—
Asst. Nurses	Units	—	—	—	—
Rented Space	(000 sq. ft)	—	—	—	—

Notes: (1) Enrollment Plan Drive.
        (2) Includes principal and capital charges over 5 years.

TABLE 25
Health Care Organization Cumulative Requirements by Quarter (Continued)

| | | | | | Practitioners | | |
| | START–UP | | | | SHAKE DOWN | | |
5	6	7	8	9 (1)	10	11	12
1800	1800	1800	1800	6300	6300	6300	6300
5400	5400	5400	5400	900	900	900	900
7200	7200	7200	7200	7200	7200	7200	7200
1/4	1/4	1/4	1/4	1/4	1/4	1/4	1/4
1/4	1/4	1/4	1/4	1/4	1/4	1/4	1/4
10	10	5.6	—	—	—	—	—
270	440	600	600	600	600	600	600
130	130	130	130	130	130	130	130
360	375	388	403	405	406	408	410
3/4	3/4	3/4	3/4	3/4	3/4	3/4	3/4
3/4	3/4	3/4	3/4	3/4	3/4	3/4	3/4
—	—	—	—	—	—	—	—
—	—	—	—	1	1	1	1
1	1	1	1	1	1	1	1
1	1	1	1	1	1	1	1
1	1	1	2	2	2	2	2
1	1	1	1	1	1	1	1
1	1	1	1	1	1	1	1
2	2	2	2	2	2	2	2
1	1	1	1	4	4	4	4
4.4	4.4	4.4	4.4	4.4	4.4	4.4	4.4
250	250	250	250	250	250	250	250
8	8	8	8	8	8	8	8
8	8	8	8	8	8	8	8
4	4	4	4	4	4	4	4
5.6	5.6	5.6	5.6	5.6	5.6	5.6	5.6

TABLE 25-2
Health Care Organization Cumulative Requirements by Quarter

ITEM	MEASURE	PRELIMINARY PLANNING 1	2	ADVANCED PLANNING 3	4
ALL UNITS					
Enrollees	Units	—	—	—	—
Other Patients	Units	—	—	—	—
Total	Units	—	—	—	—
HMO					
Adm. Director	Units	—	—	—	1/4
Clerk Secretary	Units	—	—	—	1/4
Rented Space	(000 sq. ft)	—	—	—	4.4
Building (4)	$000	—	—	—	—
Equipment (4)	$000	—	—	—	—
Systems (4)	$000	15	25	100	365
SERVICE UNIT					
Administrator	Units	—	—	—	3/4
Clerk Secretary	Units	—	—	—	3/4
Adm. Assistants	Units	—	—	—	—
Educators	Units	—	—	—	—
Asst. Doctors	Units	—	—	—	—
Head Nurses	Units	—	—	—	—
Pharmacists	Units	—	—	—	1
Lab. Technicians	Units	—	—	—	1
Radiology Tech.	Units	—	—	—	—
Bldg. Support Prsnl.	Units	—	—	—	—
Admin. Support Prsnl.	Units	—	—	—	—
Rented Space	(000 sq. ft)	—	—	—	4.4
Capital (4)	$000	—	—	—	250
MEDICAL UNIT					
Practitioners	Units	—	—	—	—
Head Nurses	Units	—	—	—	—
Asst. Nurses	Units	—	—	—	—
Rented Space	(000 sq. ft)	—	—	—	—

Notes:
(1) First Building Wing Available.
(2) Enrollment Plan Drive.
(3) Second Building Wing Available.
(4) Includes principal and capital charges over 5 years.

TABLE 25-2
Health Care Organization Cumulative Requirements by Quarter (Continued)

START-UP					16 Practitioners SHAKE DOWN		
5	6	7	8	9	10	11	12
1800	2100	2300	2600	9900	10700	11600	12600
5400	6200	6900	7600	1400	1600	1700	1800
7200	8300	9200	10200	11300	12300	13300	14400
1/4	1/4	1/4	1/4	1/4	1/4	1/4	1/4
1/4	1/4	1/4	1/4	1/4	1/4	1/4	1/4
10.0	11.7	7.7	2.8(1)	3.5	4.2	— (3)	—
390	520	650	780	910	1050	1050	1050
130	130	130	325	325	325	325	325
380	445	460	477	480	483	486	490
3/4	3/4	3/4	3/4	3/4	3/4	3/4	3/4
3/4	3/4	3/4	3/4	3/4	3/4	3/4	3/4
—	—	1	1	1	1	1	1
—	—	1	1	1	1	2	2
1	1	1	1	1	2	2	2
1	1	1	1	2	2	2	2
1	2	2	2	3	3	4	4
1	1	1	1	2	2	2	2
1	1	1	1	2	2	2	2
2	2	2	3	3	3	4	4
1	1	2	2	5	6	6	7
4.4	4.4	4.4(1)	4.4	4.4	6.3(3)	6.3	6.3
250	250	250	250	250	250	250	250
8	9	11	12	13	14	15	16
8	9	11	12	13	14	15	16
4	5	6	6	7	7	8	8
5.6	6.3	7.7	8.4	9.1	9.8	10.5	11.2

TABLE 25-3
Health Care Organization Cumulative Requirements
by Quarter

ITEM	MEASURE	PRELIMINARY PLANNING		ADVANCED PLANNING	
		1	2	3	4
ALL UNITS					
Enrollees	Units	—	—	—	—
Other Patients	Units	—	—	—	—
Total	Units	—	—	—	—
HMO					
Adm. Director	Units	—	—	—	1/4
Clerk Secretary	Units	—	—	—	1/4
Rented Space	(000 sq. ft)	—	—	—	4.4
Building (4)	$000	—	—	—	—
Equipment (4)	$000	—	—	—	—
Systems (4)	$000	15	25	195	385
SERVICE UNIT					
Administrator	Units	—	—	—	3/4
Clerk Secretary	Units	—	—	—	3/4
Adm. Assistants	Units	—	—	—	—
Educators	Units	—	—	—	—
Asst. Doctors	Units	—	—	—	—
Head Nurses	Units	—	—	—	—
Pharmacists	Units	—	—	—	1
Lab. Technicians	Units	—	—	—	1
Radiology Tech.	Units	—	—	—	—
Bldg. Support Prsnl.	Units	—	—	—	—
Adm. Support Prsnl.	Units	—	—	—	—
Rented Space	(000 sq. ft)	—	—	—	4.4
Capital (4)	$000	—	—	—	190
MEDICAL UNIT					
Practitioners	Units	—	—	—	—
Head Nurses	Units	—	—	—	—
Asst. Nurses	Units	—	—	—	—
Rented Space	(000 sq. ft)	—	—	—	—

Notes: (1) First Building Wing Available.
       (2) Enrollment Plan Drive
       (3) Second Building Wing Available.
       (4) Includes principal and capital charges over 5 years.

TABLE 25-3
Health Care Organization Cumulative Requirements
by Quarter (Continued)

					24 Practitioners		
	START-UP				SHAKE DOWN		
5	6	7	8	9(2)	10	11	12
1800	2300	2800	3400	13400	15300	17160	18900
5400	7000	8500	10000	2000	2200	2400	2700
7200	9300	11300	13400	15400	17500	19500	21600
1/4	1/4	1/4	1/4	1/4	1/4	1/4	1/4
1/4	1/4	1/4	1/4	1/4	1/4	1/4	1/4
10.0	11.4	8.4	4.2(1)	5.6	7.0	3.5(3)	5.6
520	650	780	910	1040	1170	1300	1500
130	130	130	225	225	225	325	325
415	435	454	474	478	482	486	490
3/4	3/4	3/4	3/4	3/4	3/4	3/4	3/4
3/4	3/4	3/4	3/4	3/4	3/4	3/4	3/4
—	1	1	1	1	2	2	2
—	1	1	1	2	2	2	2
1	1	1	1	2	3	3	3
1	1	1	1	2	3	3	3
1	2	2	2	3	4	5	6
1	1	1	2	2	3	3	3
1	1	1	2	2	3	3	3
2	2	2	3	3	4	4	5
1	1	2	3	7	8	9	10
4.4	4.4	4.4(1)	4.4	4.4	6.3(3)	6.3	6.3
250	250	250	250	250	250	250	250
8	10	12	14	16	18	21	24
8	10	12	14	16	18	21	24
4	5	6	7	8	9	11	12
5.6	7.0	8.4	9.8	10.2	12.6	14.7	16.8

TABLE 26
Health Care Organization Capital Requirements
5 Years

ITEM	PRACTITIONERS		
	8	16	24
LAND & BUILDINGS:			
Base Cost	520	910	1300
Capital Charge	80	140	200
Total Cost	600	1050	1500
EQUIPMENT:			
Base Cost	104	180	260
Capital Charge	26	50	65
Total Cost	130	230	325
SYSTEMS:			
Base Cost	215	230	255
Capital Charge	195	210	235
Total Cost	410	440	490
WORKING CAPITAL:			
Paid In	130	130	130
Capital Charge	120	120	120
Total Cost	250	250	250
TOTALS:			
Base Cost of Assets	969	1450	1945
Capital Charges	421	520	620
Total Cost	1390	1970	2565
COLLATERAL:			
Land & Buildings	80	140	200
Equipment	26	50	65
Systems	195	210	235
Working Capital	120	120	120
Total	421	520	620

Appendix B
Planning Case

ABOUT THE PLANNING CASE

The following plan was created in 1972 by a team of consultants and physicians with the collaboration of the HEW Regional Office in New York City. The planning procedure followed in the case was similar to that described in this handbook.

The plan was largely generated from data gathered on the job, pertaining to the neighborhood and the practices involved in the plan. Planning tables similar to those presented in Appendix A were used in the process to fill in some of the gaps.

Planning tables were also used to generate a "canned plan" to compare with the tailor-made one. As expected, it pointed up errors and inconsistencies that were corrected. The "canned plan" was remarkably like the tailor-made one except for several features that departed significantly from those assumed in the tables—notably, the center was to be an HMO requiring much more solicitation and patient recruitment than the tables assume.

PLAN FOR CREATING A COMPREHENSIVE CARE CENTER

HIGHTSTOWN MEDICAL ORGANIZATION

1972

Background

Hightstown Medical Organization is a nonprofit corporation of New Jersey created to provide comprehensive health services to residents of East Windsor Township, Hightstown Borough and surrounding communities. It is headquartered on One Mile Road Extension, Hightstown, New Jersey 08520.

A major endeavor of Hightstown Medical Organization is to create a modern health delivery system through a comprehensive health care center. This endeavor is being conducted in a special project called Hightstown Project.

The area which is now East Windsor Township and Hightstown Borough was originally settled in the early 1700s. One of the first residents was John Hight for whom the borough was named. He purchased a 3,000-acre tract along Old York Road in 1721 and established a homestead for his family near the present center of Hightstown.

The area grew slowly as a farming community until 1832 when the Camden-Amboy Railroad was constructed. This first railroad in New Jersey sparked new industry and increased the growth of the community. Hightstown Borough, in the center of East Windsor Township, was established in 1853 by an act of the legislature. It encompassed 800 acres, roughly its present size.

A map of East Windsor-Hightstown is shown as Exhibit 1. Located approximately 15 miles north of Trenton, six miles east of Princeton and 50 miles south of New York, the area lies along Route 33 connecting Trenton and Freehold, and Route 571 connecting Hightstown with Princeton. Route 539 connects Cranbury and other communities to the north. U.S. 130 and the New Jersey Turnpike pass through the area north-south, and U.S. 1 is a few miles west. East Windsor Township completely surrounds Hightstown Borough, and the two together have approximately sixteen square miles.

From a census of 2,643 in the year 1900, the population of East Windsor-Hightstown increased at a steady 600 to 650 per decade until 1960 when 6,615 people resided there. In the ten years from 1960 to 1970, the population exploded from 6,615 to approximately 16,000, an increase of 12% per year. The area is still growing rapidly. The East Windsor Township master plan, approved in December 1971, projects the population to 75,000 between the years 1990 and 2020.

Exhibit 2 is a projection of population using the master plan as a reference. Total population is projected from a present 17,000 to 35,000 in 1980 and to 56,000 in 1990. The under-age 21 group is expected to grow from 6,800 to 20,000 in 1990, the age 21-64 group from 9,600 to 32,000 and the over-age 65 group from 600 to 4,000. The medically needy group, now estimated at 500, is projected to be 2,000, while the number of self-sufficient residents goes from 16,500 to approximately 54,000 in 1990.

EXHIBIT 1
Geographic Area Served by
Hightstown Medical Organization

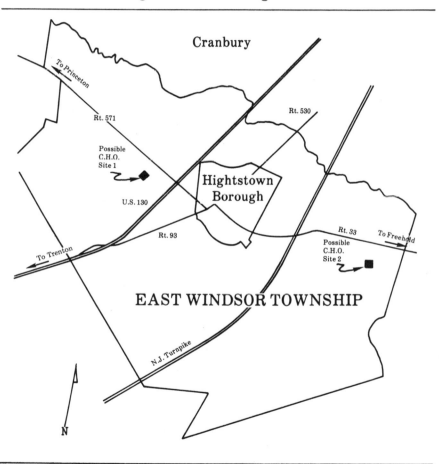

EXHIBIT 2
Estimated Population
East Windsor Township

Population by age group	Present	1980	1990
0-20	6,800	13,500	20,000
21-64	9,600	20,000	32,000
65-Over	600	1,500	4,000
Total	17,000	35,000	56,000
Self sufficient	16,500	34,000	54,000
Medically needy*	500	1,000	2,000

Notes: *Figures exclude over 65 O. A. A. recipients.
Throughout this presentation, Hightstown Borough
is included in figures identified as "East Windsor
Township."

These population figures apply to East Windsor-Hightstown only. Other nearby communities like Cranbury and Rossmoor are not included. However, for the purpose of this presentation, all of these communities will be considered in the planning, and will be designated as the East Windsor medical market.

In summation, East Windsor is relatively small, with a dense, rapidly growing population. The proportion of elderly people is low. The area is prosperous with few medically needy residents.

Preliminary investigation indicates that health status of East Windsor is comparable to that of similar communities in the United States. Exhibit 3 presents estimates of physical disorders in East Windsor,

EXHIBIT 3
Estimated Prevalence of Physical Disorder
East Windsor Township (population 17,000)

Type of Physical Disorder	Number of People Ill At a Given Time
Chronic obesity	3,000
Nervous tension	2,400
Muscles, joints & bones	1,200
Heart	1,000
Hypertension	800
Alcoholism	800
Diabetes	800
Other blood disorders	700
Psychiatric disorders	400
Urological disorders	300
Liver disorders	200
Pulmonary disorders	200
Drug addiction	200
Venereal disease	100
Other long term disorders	900
Total long term disorders	13,000
Acute illness	900
Accident recumbents	200
Pregnancy	400
Infant illness (under 1 year)	500
Total physical disorders	15,000

compiled by applying national statistics to the local population distribution.

The area has twenty physicians in full or part time residence. Medical specialties include internal medicine, gynecology, urology, ophthalmology, and pediatrics. There are two general practitioners and five surgeons. Nine dentists practice in the area. There are three pharmacies and three nursing homes, one that is a 90-bed extended care facility.

Eight hospitals are close enough to serve the area:

Princeton-six miles distant
  Princetion Hospital
Trenton-fifteen miles distant
  Hamilton Hospital   Mercer Hospital
  Helene Fuld Hospital St. Francis Hospital
Freehold-fifteen miles distant
  Freehold Area Hospital
New Brunswick- eighteen miles distant
  Middlesex General Hospital
  St. Peters Hospital

Estimates of health services provided in East Windsor, also interpolated from national statistics, are summarized in Exhibit 4. Annual cost of providing these services is estimated to be $4,500,000. This cost excludes such items as cost of psychiatric and tuberculosis care, medical education and research, and public health administration.

DEFICIENCIES IN HEALTH CARE

Even though the area is endowed with health resources. East Windsor is actually underserved from a medical viewpoint. While it does not qualify as underserved by HEW, it has what Secretary Richardson referred to as a "...non-system, cottage industry, pushcart..." medical industry.

The cost of care is rising, hospitals have unused wings and waiting lists for patients at the same time, people have difficulty in getting a physician, and preventive care is just beginning. Many citizens with health insurance have little protection against catastrophic incidents.

The critical deficiencies in health care, which President Nixon pointed out in his 1971 annual message, are problems in East Windsor just as they are in other parts of the country. The area has the resources, but does not have the system for delivering adequate care.

A survey conducted for the township master plan of 1971 indicated that the number one concern of citizens is lack of medical care. There is inadequate preventive care. While many of the more progressive physicians stress preventive care, curative care and crisis medicine are practiced to the exclusion of well-rounded comprehensive care.

EXHIBIT 4
Estimated Annual Health Services in 1971
East Windsor Township

Incident	Number	Cost (000)
Deliveries	500	$ 150
Major surgery	250	200
Minor surgery	750	100
Physician visits	70,000	800
Dental visits	20,000	300
Prescription drugs	80,000	400
Clinical tests	120,000	150
X-rays (excluding dental)	10,000	150
Short term hospital days*	20,000	1,600
ECF days	10,000	200
Prosthetics & medical supplies		100
Psychotherapy		100
Physical therapy		150
Related fiscal services		100
Total cost of health incidents		$4,500**

Notes: *   Excludes inpatient tests, drugs, operating room costs, anesthesia, and therapy.

     **   Excludes long-term care in state institutions, custodial care, and other services of a general nature amounting to an estimated $1,100,000.

Based on preliminary impressions, chronic illness susceptible to preventive care is as much a problem in East Windsor as in other sections of the country. Health education programs, periodic health examinations, and a family health monitoring system are needed. Some of the medical services which are not adequate include:

>Preventive medical care such as —
>>Periodic physical examination
>>Complete problem-oriented medical histories
>>Well-child care
>Immunization programs
>Medical education, including family planning
>Home health care and other outreach services
>Emergency care away from hospital
>Environmental protection, including prevention of communicable diseases
>Alcohol and drug therapy

The physicians of Hightstown Medical Organization practice preventive medicine. They give periodic physical examinations, keep medical histories, and use multi-phasic screening in diagnosis. However, they are limited in time and resources. As the new organization develops, they plan to increase physical examinations, automate medical histories, utilize more testing procedures, and employ paramedics. The accomplishment of these objectives will take time, require additional personnel, and probably a new system of care.

A rough estimate of the cost of medical care in East Windsor interpolated from national statistics is shown as Exhibit 5. Cost of premature death in lost productive power is estimated at $3,000,000 annually, cost of absenteeism from work at $4,000,000, inefficiency resulting from debilitative disorders at $3,500,000, and cost of medical treatment at $4,500,000. The total cost of $15,000,000 annually is almost $1,000 per year for every person in the area.

These statistics exclude the grief and unhappiness which accompany ill health. And while they are rough estimates, they indicate the magnitude of the medical problems in a community that is well endowed.

OPPORTUNITIES

Most states, including New Jersey, have passed enabling legislation for establishment of HMOs. In 48 of the states, physicians are permit-

---

EXHIBIT 5
Estimated Cost of Illness in 1971
East Windsor Township

Premature mortality	$ 3,000,000
Absenteeism	4,000,000
Inefficiency	3,500,000
Cost of treatment*	4,500,000
Total cost of illness	15,000,000

Note: *Excludes cost of long-term care in
hospitals and other institutions.

---

ted to incorporate, and thereby attain tax advantages previously not available to them. In addition to opportunities afforded by federal and state legislation, there are local opportunities for a better health delivery system. East Windsor is a well endowed area. The residents are educated and progressive in their thinking. Population density is high and going higher. The community has a small number of elderly people as well as medically indigent. It is strong enough to develop a comprehensive care system without large subsidies.

There is a desire among some physicians in the area to improve the system. But most important, East Windsor has the resources for a successful health care center, including:

1. The necessary primary care physicians.
2. Sufficient dentists and pharmacists to serve the community.
3. Eight hospitals near enough to provide inpatient care.
4. Specialist services within comparatively short driving distance.
5. Progressive local government and citizens concerned with health care.

6. Two new medical facilities recently completed, ideally located to provide medical care.

7. Medical providers willing to cooperate in the development of an ideal system.

In summation, currently available resources, local attitudes, and an ideally suited community make the prospect of creating a successful health care center in the near future feasible and highly probable.

HIGHTSTOWN PROJECT

Seeing the need and opportunity, sponsors of Hightstown Medical Organization created the Hightstown Project to improve the medical delivery system in the area. The project team was charged with exploring the feasibility of a comprehensive health care organization (CHO), for planning one, if feasible, and for subsequent development, if the proposed system were desirable.

Accomplishments to Date

Conceptual planning of the project has been completed. A conclusion has been reached that creation of a CHO in East Windsor is feasible, desirable, and would have a reasonable probability of success. Discussions have been held with prospective sponsors, providers, community leaders, and representatives of federal and state agencies. Everyone contacted has expressed willingness to cooperate in the venture.

The objectives of the project have been formulated and summarized. They call for early creation of a health care system in accordance with guidelines issued by HEW.

A system plan has been devised and summarized. It gives an overall description and details of organization, internal operating systems, control systems, physical facilities, and fiscal operations.

Finally, a project program has been formulated to develop plans, construct facilities, start up operations, and monitor the system in its early operations.

Most of the tasks in HEW's guidelines for phases I and II of the HMO evolvement have been completed. Financial, consumer, and medical care resources have been analyzed and the potential market for services determined. Community leadership and potential partners have been partly identified. Specifications have been established for control systems, including a linked data system and a system to monitor effectiveness of the project.

The Hightstown Medical Organization has been incorporated as a nonprofit organization to provide medical services in East Windsor. It will be modified to conform with DHEW requirements for HMOs. Arrangements are being explored with hospitals and other institutional providers of medical care.

A tentative benefits package and a prepayment plan have been roughed out. Discussions are under way with potential fiscal intermediaries for the prepayment program.

Health care goals have been tentatively established, and capital needs for development, facilities construction, and a program to start-up have been estimated.

Necessary dialogues with cognizant agencies at the federal and state levels have been started. The reaction of the state comprehensive planning agency is attached to this report.

What Remains to be Done

There is much to be done. Several of the initial planning tasks need to be completed. For example, key personnel need to be employed, including a full-time director. Commitments of enrollee groups must be sought at an early date. To accomplish this, a program of education and indoctrination must be implemented as early as possible. Draft contracts between the HMO and its component parts, now being considered by legal counsel, need to be completed.

The immediate task is to get an advanced planning program under way. Plans should be refined and developed with emphasis on receiving and utilizing inputs from citizen representatives and provider groups.

Working relationships with public agencies need to be formalized; legal research is required to evaluate the critical constraints identified in planning; and as many medical providers should be lined up as soon as possible.

Further planning work will include:

1. Refining the initial prepayment package.
2. Further search for a potential fiscal intermediary.
3. Initial negotiations of enrollee contracts.
4. Recruitment of potential enrollees.
5. Finalization of the HMO organization.
6. Design of operating and control systems.
7. Design of facilities and equipment required.

After the advanced planning phase, the initial staffing and construction phase must be completed. Equipment and supplies need to be procured, renovation accomplished. Key personnel must be recruited and trained and enrollment of users started.

Finally, the start-up phase needs to be initiated. This will consist of actively recruiting enrollees, hiring support personnel, installing new systems, commencing and shaking down operations.

REQUEST FOR FUNDS

A request has been made to secure $170,000 in federal funds, under PL89-749 Section 314(e), to conduct advance planning work. It is believed that the funds will enable Hightstown Medical Organization to do the planning work in six months.

Since most of the facilities needed are available, it will be possible to perform the initial staffing and construction phase in a short period and even to overlap this work to some degree with start-up operations. Thus, it is feasible to complete the overall project in one year, a goal which has been adopted. The funds sought should pave the way to that goal; without them, the program would be stymied.

In addition to financing development, the grant will demonstrate a unique approach to an HMO. Plans envision creation of an effective center, not only in a short time, but with a minimum of federal funds. By an evolutionary approach, existing physician practices will be brought together, reshaped, and realigned to meet the specifications of an HMO without need for large operational subsidies.

The plan allows for mixing fee-for-service patients with pre-payers as it evolves to a full prepayment status. This feature alone makes the plan acceptable to providers and users who would otherwise reject it. It also keeps the break-even cost below that of other more touted approaches, making the center self-sufficient with but a small number of prepaid enrollees.

In short, the funds requested will make possible creation of a health delivery system that could be a model for other suburban communities in the country.

OBJECTIVES

The objective of the Hightstown Project is to create a comprehensive medical care system in the greater East Windsor area to improve the health of inhabitants at the lowest practical cost.

The heart of the system will be the Hightstown Medical Organization, functioning as a comprehensive health care center to provide enrollees with medical services — inhouse and by outside medical providers working under provider contracts.

The proposed system should prevent disease, extend life, make enrollees more useful and increase their capacity to enjoy life. While it is difficult to measure progress toward such goals, effort will be made to do so with techniques available.

A concerted effort will be made to reduce the numbers of disorders shown in Exhibit 3. Exhibit 6 is a preliminary list of medical case goals for 1980. These goals, while subject to refinement, target a reduction of disorders in East Windsor of about one-third — or two-thirds of what could be expected under the present system. Sizable inroads on illness are expected as the result of enrollee education, periodic physical examinations, improved medical records, environmental protection, alcohol and drug therapy, and other health services.

There is evidence that obesity, nervous tension, heart disorders, and related illnesses can be reduced through preventive care involving nutrition, exercise, and mental conditioning. Inroads can be made on hypertension, anemia, chronic nephritis, and arthritis, for example, through early detection and treatment. While alcoholism and other addictive diseases cannot be cured, they can be arrested by proper treatment and prevented, to a degree, through proper education.

Early cancer can frequently be detected and cured. Working closely with research organizations and teaching facilities, the proposed system would have an effective program of cancer detection.

Acute illnesses should be reduced as chronic illness declines. It should also decline with immunization, environmental protection, and general health conditioning.

Through a family health monitoring system, unwanted pregnancies, veneral disease, and preventable diseases should be reduced. Epidemiological statistics should be kept in coordination with the state department of public health to detect and prevent the onslaught of communicable diseases, and to trace diseases to environmental sources.

Finally, a program of dental care for children will reduce care required when the children become adults.

The medical goals spelled out in Exhibit 6 need refinement. Indeed, they should be challenged not only at the start, but periodically, as the

EXHIBIT 6
Disease Prevalence Goals for 1980
East Windsor Township
(Projected population 34,000)

Disorders	Number of People Ill at a Given Time	
	Present System	New System
Obesity	6,000	3,000
Nervous Tension	4,800	3,400
Muscles, joints & bones	2,400	1,500
Heart	2,000	1,500
Hypertension	1,600	1,200
Alcoholism, active	1,600	800
Diabetes	1,600	1,600
Other blood disorders	1,400	1,200
Psychiatric disorders	800	500
Urological disorders	600	400
Liver disorders	400	300
Pulmonary disorders	400	200
Drug addiction, active	400	100
Venereal disease	200	100
Other long term disorders	1,800	1,200
Total long term disorders	26,000	17,000
Acute illnesses	1,800	1,200
Accident recumbents	400	400
Pregnancy cases	800	800
Infant illnesses (under 1 year)	1,000	1,000
Total medical cases	30,000	20,400

program develops. It is expected that initial goals will be raised as time passes.

In establishing goals, consideration should be given to economic trade-offs. For example, there is a point of dimishing return regarding most tests and procedures. Since these points do not follow specific rules, medical judgment supported by the latest evidence should be used to strike the optimum balance between prevention, cure, and cost. This judgment must be exercised to establish realistic long-run goals.

Once case goals have been established, service goals should follow. Reductions in illnesses should be accompanied by fewer physician visits, fewer hospital days, and reduced need for drugs. Exhibit 7 presents tentative health service goals for 1980. These goals also need periodic revision and refinement. Tentatively at least, the services rendered are targeted ten percent lower in the proposed system than under the present one extended.

Overall economic goals are presented in Exhibit 8. Life should be extended through better medical care, absenteeism reduced and human efficiency increased. Together with a reduction in medical service costs, the proposed system is targeted to reduce the overall cost of illness by 1980 by some $5,000,000. These goals are stated in rough figures which must be revised and refined periodically.

Finally, the capacity to enjoy life through better health should be significantly improved. While there are no direct indicators for this goal, there is an obvious correlation between reduction of illness and life enjoyment. It is safe to assume that intangible gains are related to economic gains, and should far surpass them in social value as general health is improved.

Medical Services

The proposed system will consist of primary medical services including:

Enrollee education,
Patient health audit,
Physician care,
Surgical care,
Dental care,
Institutional care,
Prescription drugs,
Therapy, and
Immunization.

EXHIBIT 7
Annual Health Services Goals for 1980
East Windsor Township
(Projected population 34,000)

Incidents	Projected Cost (000) (constant $s)	
	Present System	New System
Deliveries	$ 300	$ 300
Major surgery	400	350
Minor surgery	200	150
Physician visits (a)	1,600	1,200
Dental visits	600	600
Prescription drugs (a)	800	500
Clinical tests (a)	300	500
X-ray (excluding dental) (a)	300	400
Short term hospital days (b)	3,200	2,000
Extended care (b)	400	600
Prosthetics & medical supplies	200	200
Psychotherapy	200	300
Physical therapy (b)	300	200
Education		200
Environmental protection		200
Related fiscal services	200	300
Total costs	$9,000	$8,000

Notes: (a) Includes preventive medical care at an estimated cost of
$250,000 under "present system" and $700,000
under the "new system."

(b) Includes private duty nursing, home health care and
similar categories of medical care. Table excludes
long-term care in state institutions, custodial care,
and other services of a general nature amounting to
an estimated $2,200,000.

EXHIBIT 8
Medical Economic Goals For 1980
East Windsor Township
(Projected population 34,000)

	Projected Costs (constant $s)	
	Present System	New System
Premature mortality	$ 6,000,000	$ 5,000,000
Absenteeism	8,000,000	6,000,000
Inefficiency	7,000,000	6,000,000
Cost of treatment*	9,000,000	8,000,000
Total cost of illness	$30,000,000	$25,000,000

Note* Excludes cost of long-term care in hospitals and other institutions.

These services will be administered to prevent disease, to arrest it, to cure patients and to rehabilitate them following serious disorders. Exhibit 9 is a table of primary services and the purposes of them.

Education programs for enrollees will be continuous to cover a range of subjects including: family planning, disease prevention, exercise, diet and nutrition, importance of physical examinations, how to detect physical disorders, well baby care, geriatrics, immunization programs, mental health, and others.

In addition, courses will be given on the nature of disease, how to adjust to it, and how to understand and follow physicians' orders.

Patient health audits will include periodic physical examinations, maintenance of medical history records, and followup treatment. Physical examinations will be scheduled according to age, sex, and health of an individual. The frequency and composition of health screens will be tailored to groups of enrollees. For example, the elderly and ill will be screened more frequently than the young and healthy. Special tests will be given to those known to have or suspected of having a chronic disorder.

EXHIBIT 9
Proposed Primary Services by Purpose

Benefits	Purpose			
	Disorder Prevention	Disorder Cure	Rehabilitative Care	Disease Arrestment
Enrollee education	X	X	X	X
Patient health audit	X	X		
Physician care of:				
Baby	X	X	X	X
Mother	X	X	X	X
Other	X	X		
Dental care	X	X	X	
Drugs	X	X	X	X
Therapy				
Physical		X	X	X
Psychiatric		X	X	
Immunization	X			
Institutional care		X	X	X

Physician care will be given for all purposes, including prevention of disease. Included will be well baby care, pre- and post-natal care of mothers, and general and specialty care of others. Physicians will counsel patients, examine them, prescribe tests, make diagnoses, prescribe treatment, administer general therapy, follow up on treatment and see that the patient is properly handled.

Surgical care will be provided, including major and minor procedures. While limitations will be applied to the prepayment package, every available kind of surgery will at least be available for a fee.

Dental care will also be provided, including dental surgery, orthodonture, preventive series, root canal work, and dentures. Care will be available either in-house or by outside dental providers, with other than limited care provided on a fee-for-service basis.

Institutional care will be provided, including care in a hospital or extended care facility; also use of operating facilities, anesthesia, and other services generally rendered by a medical institution will be provided.

Prescription drugs will be provided. Vitamins and other pharmaceuticals will be available for a fee.

Physical and psychiatric therapy will be provided either inhouse or by outside providers. Alcoholic and drug therapy will be available but only therapy deemed essential by a physician will be included in the prepayment package.

Immunization will be provided, including infant and child inoculations and special series to combat epidemics.

These services will be provided at inhouse care centers at outside provider premises, and at patients' homes. Five primary care centers will be established inhouse: for education, diagnostic support, emergency care, practitioner care, and drug distribution. Exhibit 10 illustrates how primary services will be distributed among care centers. It also shows whether care is administered inhouse or by an out of house provider under contract.

EXHIBIT 10
Proposed Primary Services by Care Center

	Care Centers							
Primary Services	Education	Diagnostic	Emergency	Practitioners	Drug Dispensary	Hospital	ECF	Patient's Home
Patient Education	H							
Patient health audit		H&C						
Physician care of:								
Baby			H&C	H&C		C		H
Mother			H&C	H&C		C	C	H
Other			H&C	H&C		C	C	H
Dental care			H&C	H&C				
Drugs					H	C	C	
Therapy:								
Physical				H&C		C	C	H&C
Psychiatric				H&C		C	C	
Immunization				H				
Institutional care						C	C	

Notes: H - Care inhouse
       C - Contract provider care out-of-house

Enrollee education, for example, will be conducted in a house educational center. Patient health audits will be done in a house diagnostic center using house and outside laboratory facilities. General care and some specialty care will be rendered in practitioner centers, the emergency center, institutions, and patients' homes, while most specialty care will be given under contract on the premises of specialists. Dental care will be administered inhouse and by contract providers out of house.

Institutional care will be purchased by contract in the institution concerned. Pharmaceuticals will be dispensed inhouse and by insitutions under contract. Therapy will be rendered inhouse and by outside providers.

In addition to primary care, the following major support services will be provided for inhouse care centers:

> Laboratory services,
> Diagnostic X-ray,
> Transportation,
> Medical supplies,
> Facilities support,
> Staff training,
> Data processing, and
> Administrative support.

Some of these will be provided by house employees; others by outside contractors. Exhibit 11 lists the support services, the care centers they serve, and whether provided inhouse or by the outside.

For example, laboratory services and diagnostic X-ray will be furnished to the diagnostic center, emergency center, and practitioners both by house facilities and by outside suppliers. Ambulance service will be provided by outsiders to enrollees between homes, the emergency center, and institutions. Mini-bus and auto transportation will be provided all care centers by house facilities. Supplies, facilities support, and data processing will be provided to all house centers by inside and outside providers. Staff training will be provided to all care centers by a house staff. Administrative support will be provided by the house to all care centers in the system.

Benefit Packages

In addition to a full range of medical services, the center will offer prepayment benefit packages, payable by enrollees, their employers, cognizant government agencies, and others.

EXHIBIT 11
Proposed Support Services by Care Center

SERVICES	Education	Diagnostics	Emergency	Practitioners	Drug Dispensary	Hospital	Other Care Facilities	Patient's Home
					CARE CENTERS SERVED			
Laboratory Services		h,c	h,c	h,c				
Diagnostic X-ray (excluding dental)		h,c	h,c	h,c				
Transportation								
ambulance	c					c	c	c
minibus	h	h	h	h		h	h	
autopool	h	h	h	h	h	h	h	h
Medical Supplies	h,c	h,c	h,c	h,c	h,c	h,c		
Facility Support	h,c	h,c	h,c	h,c	h,c	h,c		
Staff Training	h	h	h	h	h	h		
Data Processing	h,c	h,c	h,c	h,c	h,c			
Administrative Support	h	h	h	h	h	h	h	h

Legend: h — provided inhouse
       c — contractor provided

Tentatively, the packages will include basic services and add-ons for prescription drugs, dental care and other options. Following guidelines of Secretary Richardson, the payment plans will have annual premiums with deductibles and coinsurance provisions.

The tentative basic package will include:

1. Hospital care or care in an extended care facility.
2. Essential surgery, use of operating rooms, anesthesia, etc.
3. Pre- and post-natal care and delivery.
4. Physician visits, including well baby care.
5. Home health care.
6. Essential therapy.
7. Preventive care, including health audits and inoculations.
8. Emergency care on a 24-hour basis.
9. Ambulance service as needed.

Exhibit 12 presents a tentative prepayment package for enrollees up to age 65 who are not covered by Medicaid. A similar package will be developed for Medicare and Medicaid enrollees.

An annual premium of approximately $130 per person is anticipated with a deductible of $75 per person per year and coinsurance of 25%, not to exceed $1500 annually per family. A rider of approximately $20 per person per year will be considered to cover prescription drugs and one of $20 to cover preventive dental care. It must be noted that these are planning figures subject to revision as information is generated about the health status of the covered population.

It is planned to use a fiscal intermediary to collect premiums and distribute funds to the center on a capitation basis, estimated at approximately $270 per person per year for all coverage, including copayments.

Preliminary actuarial analysis indicates that a relatively large number of enrollees are needed to make the payment plan feasible. There are normal variations where an individual incurs up to several thousand dollars' expense in a year and catastrophic variations where he incurs $10,000 to $50,000 or more. The normal variations are smoothed sufficiently with 3,000 or more enrollees; the catastrophe variations are smoothed with 12,000 or more; both variations together with 20,000 or more. Variations in cost of care for different enrollment levels are presented in Exhibit 13.

To assure orderly payment under the prepayment plan, at least 3,000 must be enrolled with catastrophic insurance for all enrollees. This should keep chance variation in any one year to 13% or less. To

---

EXHIBIT 12
Tentative Initial Prepayment Package

Services Offered	Enrollee Expenditure (cost per person)

1. Basic package

    inpatient hospital care

    ECF care

    major and minor surgery, including anesthesia & necessary X-ray

    obstetrics, including prenatal and postnatal care for mother and baby

    physician care, including well-child care

    home health care as needed

    essential therapy

    preventive care, including health audits and inoculations

    health education, including environmental protection

    emergency care on 24 hour basis

    ambulance service

    out of area medical care as necessary

    annual premium: $130 per person

    deductibles: $75
    copay: 25% over $75

    total cost not to exceed $1500 per year per family

2. Prescription drugs   annual premium: $20

3. Dental care

    preventive care and routine curative care for children (2 visits per year)   annual premium: $20

4. Necessary physician house calls

    day-time calls $5 per visit

    night-time calls $10 per visit

Note: These services and tentative cost figures would be available to all enrollees up to age 65 who are not recipients of Medicaid.

---

further reduce fluctuation risks, the fiscal plan must provide that deficits and surpluses due to chance variations be shared by the center, providers in the plan, and the fiscal intermediary.

EXHIBIT 13
Estimated Maximum Variation in Cost of Care
(based on P = .001)

Enrollees	Total Cost (000)	Normal Variations		Catastrophe Variations	
		±000	% total	±000	% total
1	$ 0.25	$ 1.4	560%	$ 25	10,000%
10	2.50	8.4	336	25	1,000
100	25.00	36.0	144	50	200
200	50.00	45.0	90	75	150
400	100.00	55.0	55	110	110
800	200.00	66.0	33	132	66
1,600	400.00	80.0	20	160	40
3,200	800.00	100.0	13	200	26
6,400	1,600.00	128.0	8	256	16
12,800	3,200.00	160.0	5	320	10
25,600	6,400.00	200.0	3	400	6
51,200	12,800.00	280.0	2	560	4
102,400	25,600.00	400.00	1.5	800	3

Assumptions:

1. Catastrophe case frequency of .001 at $25,000 cost per case.
2. High normal year frequency of 0.1 at $1,400 per year per enrollee.

Special Features

Emergency services will be provided around the clock, other services available from 9 to 5 on a continuing weekday basis. Services will be of high quality, insured by quality controls. They will be available to everyone, regardless of race, creed, or color. Open enrollment will be held at least once every year for persons in the community.

Emphasis will be given to disease prevention, outreach, and family health management. To make sure enrollees are satisfied, their views will be sought by representation on the board of trustees.

Cost of care will be kept to a practical minimum. To achieve this, incentives to use ambulatory facilities will be adopted. Enrollees will be taught to take care of their health.

The system will be attractive to both enrollees and providers. Enrollees will be treated with dignity, and should never become financially dependent on the system. They will have a range of benefits and payment plans from which to choose. If they are out of town, provisions will be made for handling illness. Patient-doctor relationships, desired by both patients and doctors, will be preserved as far as possible in keeping with other objectives. Adequate incentives for doctors will be adopted: shorter hours of work, group consultation, service support, continued professional education, estate planning, income tax benefits, etc.

Finally, the system will be flexible, capable of growing with the community and changing mix of services to meet needs of the population.

By 1980, Hightstown Medical Organization should be capable of serving 35,000 people. Its care package should be expanded to include ultimately most health services. A large shift should take place from crisis to preventive care. Per capita cost of care should decline modestly while overall cost of disease declines a sizeable amount.

OBSTACLES

A major drawback that must be avoided in the proposed center is high start-up cost. This must be avoided if the project is to succeed.

High start-up cost is related to the kind of plan and number of enrollees. For example, if the plan calls for 100% prepayment at the start, it will need 20,000 or more enrollees to become financially independent. This is a high enrollment, and in a time of uncertainty, would be virtually impossible to achieve without enormous start-up costs. If, on the other hand, the plan approaches full prepayment in an evolutionary way, allowing a mix of fee-for-service patients with prepayment enrollees, cost of start-up could be kept low. Physicians joining the center under this plan would bring along their regular patients, serving them as usual until they elected prepayment.

Another major obstacle is physician reluctance. The American Medical Association, in a published statement on HMOs, said recently, "...many physicians prefer solo practice. These physicians are not likely to accept the HMO approach which can involve agreeing to an audit of medical practices and prorating physician fees to pay for other services. In addition, physicians are trained more for the treatment of illness than for the maintenance of health, their education is crisis oriented, and some might feel professional dissatisfaction in seeing healthy patients."

This obstacle can be overcome by incentives for physicians: better facilities, the chance to work closely with colleagues, shorter hours, planned vacations, time for self-improvement, and others. But most important, doctors are not willing to risk their present practice, take a cut in income, and work for someone else. However, they can be persuaded to join a federation that preserves their independence, rendering service on a contract basis, sharing capitation income on a fee-for-service proration. In short, they can have the best features of group and solo practice, provided the system is structured to give it to them.

A third major obstacle is the enrollee. He is not likely to join a prepayment plan until his employer assumes some of the cost. With future legislation uncertain, coupled with union interest in extending local concessions corporation-wide, industrial companies are likely to adopt a wait-and-see policy.

The answer to this problem too is the flexible approach. Allowing a mix of fee-for-service patients along with prepayers makes enrollment delays less than a catastrophe.

A final barrier is the reluctance of venture capital. Even with low start-up costs, investors are likely to be wary of medical centers unless they can get a return commensurate with risk. Once again there is an answer: the center can be structured to combine functions requiring start up capital in a profitmaking corporation. This done, venture capital can be attracted from a number of private sources.

GUIDELINES

To reach objectives and overcome obstacles, the following guidelines will be used to create the new system:

1. It will be recognized that everyone should have the opportunity to get good health care.
2. To provide good care, compromises will be made. For example, limitations will be required on initial benefit packages with the expectation that limitations can be relaxed over the years.
3. A sharp break with traditional care, which would require large start-up costs, should be avoided. The approach should be evolutionary, bringing together existing practices for progressive consolidation and realignment.

4. The uncertainty of pending legislation calls for flexible prepayment packages. For the under 65 group, packages should be based on current insurance with riders to bridge present and desired coverage, adjustable as federal guidelines are formulated.
5. The plan should be attractive to providers and users. In addition to being evolutionary, it should have other incentives to attract participants.
6. There is a reluctance of providers to make unilateral sacrifices in a prosperous community, and unless recognized, this will defeat the project. The plan, therefore, should envision economic sacrifice for no one but rely only on gains that can be achieved through better health care.
7. Excessive earnings by providers should be discouraged but not payment of fair compensation for essential resources. For example, venture capital can be attained only by a proposition which is competitive with other ventures.
8. Trade-offs should be made to preserve doctor-patient relationships, maintain professional independence, and retain coveted status. To do this, the system should be organized in a consortium bound by contracts rather than a single monolithic corporation.

In short, the guiding philosophy is to create an improved system of medical care taking the course most likely to succeed. Success is essential, and should be given emphasis with other objectives.

MEDICAL SYSTEM PLAN

The ultimate system of care will be structured around users of the system, a health care center, and contract providers outside the center. The health maintenance center, in turn, will be comprised of a plan organization, a group of medical practitioners, a medical management corporation, a fiscal intermediary, and a venture capital association. An outline of the components is shown below:

USERS   Residents of East Windsor

HMX   Health Maintenance Center:

      HMO   Hightstown Plan Organization (Plan Unit)
      HMG   Hightstown Medical Group
      HMC   Hightstown Management Corporation (Service Unit)

HFI   Hightstown Fiscal Intermediary
HCC   Hightstown Capital Corporation

OP   Outside providers

The health maintenance center (HMX) will be a federation of the five following groups tightly combined by contract:

1. HMO, a nonprofit corporation that coordinates others, buys services of providers, and sells them to enrolled users — the health plan unit of the complex.
2. HMG, a house medical group that gives primary care to enrollees.
3. HMC, a profit corporation which provides administrative and medical support services to HMO, HMG, and users.
4. HFI, a fiscal intermediary which collects from enrollees or other payers and reimburses HMO on a per capita basis.
5. HCC, a venture capital corporation which provides start-up capital.

Three of the organizations, HMO, HMG, and HMC, will share facilities, operating together in clinical fashion.

Exhibit 14 illustrates how the components will work together as a system. Services will flow from sources to users, directly in the case of outside providers and through the center in the case of house providers. Payments in turn go from payers to suppliers largely through the fiscal intermediary and party around it from patient to center.

It should be noted that the proposed flow of funds shown is based on 100% enrollment. In early stages when enrollment is small, a large part of the funds will bypass the fiscal intermediary, going directly from patient to physician.

Organization

The five component organizations of the health center will be linked by working contracts. This relationship is portrayed in Exhibit 15-1.

The plan organization, HMO, will formulate and promulgate policy governing the entire center. Its board of trustees will have providers, community leaders, consumer representatives, etc. An administrator will serve the board and see that policies are carried out. In addition to making policy, HMO will purchase services for enrollees, collect capita-

EXHIBIT 14
Overall System Configuration
Flow of Services

FLOW OF SERVICES

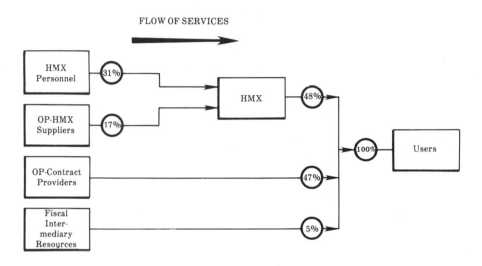

FLOW OF FUNDS

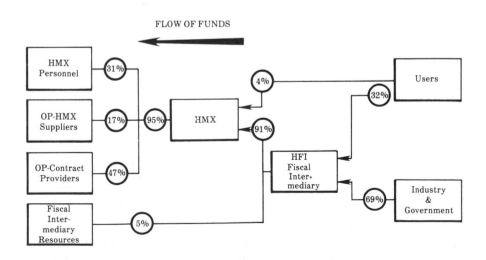

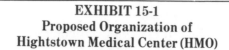

EXHIBIT 15-1
Proposed Organization of
Hightstown Medical Center (HMO)

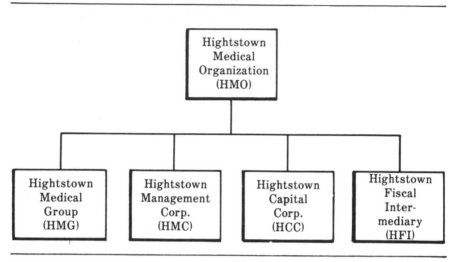

tion payments and rentals, pay contract providers, pay the management corporation and medical practitioners, and prorate its gains and losses among providers in the prepayment plan.

The management corporation, HMC, headed by a board of directors and president, will provide support services to the center: administrative services, education, diagnostic support, X-ray, drugs, building services, etc. It will also maintain the emergency facility and provide home care by visiting nurses.

The medical group, HMG, will consist of solo practitioners, partners, and practitioners organized in professional corporations. It will provide primary medical care and care of specialists who join the prepayment plan. In the beginning, the medical group will largely serve its own patients on a fee-for-service basis. As enrollment grows, it will serve progressively more enrollees. Included in the medical group will be general practitioners, internists, pediatricians, gynecologists, urologists, and other specialists.

The fiscal intermediary, HFI, a health insurance company, will market the prepayment plan, collect premiums, deductibles, co-payments and other fees from payers. It will contract for catastrophic coverage for all enrollees on a group insurance basis, keep reserves, and reimburse HMO on a capitation basis. In addition, the intermediary will advise HMO on premiums, enrollment campaigns, and areas of support. It will also make periodic audits of services rendered.

The capital association, HCC, a bank, investment company or other, will provide the capital for start-up of the management corporation.

Exhibit 15-2 is a tentative organization chart of HMC, the proposed management corporation.

The corporation will be headed by a president who will also serve as administrator of HMO. It will be a profit corporation with seven primary departments:

> Administration,
> General Services,
> Education,
> Diagnostic Center,
> X-ray,
> Emergency and Outreach Services, and
> Drug Distribution Center.

The administrative department will do the administrative support work of HMO and the management corporation, including booking, billing, bookkeeping and the maintenance of files. It will perform purchas-

---

EXHIBIT 15-2
Proposed Organization of
Management Corporation (HMC)

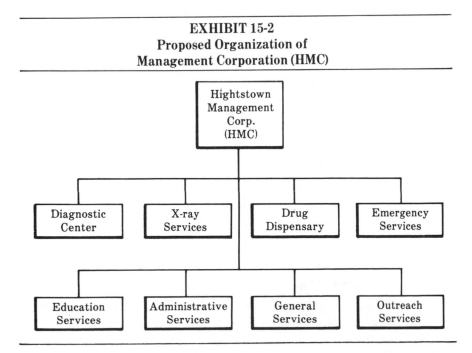

ing agent functions and make payments. On request, it will handle the paper work of house practitioners and provide them with other business services. It will be responsible for administrative aspects of enrollee health management and quality control of medical services. Finally, it will provide data processing for all departments and be responsible for the linked data system of the center.

The X-ray department will be headed by a contract provider or plan member who will be responsible for the equipment and will provide practitioners with a range of diagnostic X-ray procedures. HMC will be responsible only for the space used, the provider contract, and follow up on contract terms. As required, the X-ray department will acquire the services of other providers.

Emergency & Outreach, headed by a paramed, will manage the emergency facility and provide outreach services by visiting nurses and home health aides. The facility will be staffed by parameds who will call upon physicians and surgeons as needed. A physician will be in charge of medical affairs at all times. HMC will be responsible for space and to see that the facility is properly staffed.

General Services, headed by an administrative assistant, will provide building operation and maintenance, transportation, communication services, etc. It will acquire services of outside suppliers as needed through the administrative department.

The education department, headed by an educator, will provide enrollee education and inhouse training of medical support staffs. It will run the medical library and furnish educational aids for patients. The department will also run the environmental protection program including compilation of epidemiological data. In addition, it will handle public relations.

The diagnostic center, headed by a resident, will give periodic physical examinations to enrollees and on request to non-enrollees, and also, on request, will do special health screens for users. It will handle the medical history files of enrollees. Finally, it will operate a stat laboratory for physicians and will get laboratory services from outside as needed.

The drug dispensary, headed by a pharmacist, will fill prescriptions for enrollees and others on request. It will purchase, store, mix, package, and distribute drugs.

Organization structure prescribed is tentative. It will be refined as the center evolves. In the early stages, the structure will be kept simple, utilizing personnel as efficiently as possible.

Internal Service Systems

Particular care will be given to creation of the following internal service systems:

1. Medical education system.
2. Patient health screen system.
3. Physician services system.
4. Emergency care system.
5. Drug distribution system.
6. Patient logistics system.

Medical Education System

The medical education system will be a family of related systems; each will involve accumulation of information, its manipulation, and dissemination.

Through journals, the professional staff, medical meetings, news releases, HEW, the state department of health, universities, research organizations, and others, the department will gather information germane to health of enrollees such as new discoveries, drugs, immunization, and procedures. After sifting and checking, bulletins will be prepared and mailed to enrollees. Where information is critical, letters will be sent to enrollees through their physicians.

General bulletins will be issued on diet, exercise, sleep, relaxation, care of a cold, and others. These will be revised periodically. Emergency bulletins will be sent to warn of epidemics, environmental hazards, and availability of special injections, screening, and treatment.

Courses will be held on subjects such as family planning, physical conditioning, routine examinations for cancer, cleanliness habits, food preservation, etc. Special visual and audio presentations will be developed on a variety of subjects such as the nature of a myocardial infarction, its diagnosis, and what the patient should do in following instructions.

Other information systems will include public information, press releases, and information required by government agencies and professional organizations.

A series of training programs will be planned for paraprofessionals, support staff members, and other employees. Training aids and programs will be developed for professional employees using professional guidance.

Patient Health Screening System

A family of health screening systems will be devised with the consent and advice of house physicians. Patients will be scheduled in advance for periodic examinations. Depending upon age, sex, and physical condition, each will be assigned a series of examinations covering items such as patient history, hands-on examination, blood pressure, pulse, cardiometer, chest X-ray, audiometry, visual acuity, tonometry, spirometry, proctoscopy, pap smear, arthrometrics, and biochemical analyses. Information will be processed by automated business equipment, including a computer analysis of findings. Results will be sent to physicians for review.

In addition, special screening will be performed on request. The same general procedures will be followed, altered as necessary by physicians. Where single tests and simple series such as an SMA 12 are required, samples of blood and urine will be taken, tests run, and results forwarded to physicians. Some of these will be performed in a stat laboratory.

Physician Service System

Each physician will be responsible for his own system of dispensing services. Facilities of the center will be laid out to accommodate each one to the extent practicable.

The general practice will be patients visiting the center for medical services. They should be able to do so at all times in the emergency facility, and during office hours in the offices of practitioners. It is expected that users will choose their primary care physicians, who will refer them to specialists as needed.

Medical services will be rendered in the emergency facility as required. This may make a physician leave his offices temporarily to render treatment. Services will also be provided in hospitals, extended care facilities, and in patients' homes.

Parameds or assistant doctors will be encouraged to relieve physicians and keep cost of service down. Sharing of facilities, like examining rooms, and of personnel, such as nurses, will be urged to keep costs down. While each physician will have the choice of keeping his own records, HMC will install booking, billing, and bookkeeping systems to serve physicians who may desire them. A joint switchboard, telephone operator, and receptionist will be available to all practitioners.

Emergency Care System

The emergency care system will handle patients who require immediate attention, and those who can be treated by simple procedures. Accidents, seizures, and minor illnesses will be treated in the facility as decided by patients and attending physicians. In severe emergencies, life-saving procedures, such as heart defibrilation, will be administered, and patients will be kept overnight if moving them to a hospital jeopardizes their health.

Generally, patients will transport themselves to the center for emergency treatment. If necessary, transportation will be provided, including ambulance service.

The emergency facility will operate on a 24-hour basis with a flexible duty staff backed by a standby staff. Within defined guidelines, it will provide a range of staff services from nurse to surgeon. The facility will be under the supervision of a physician at all times.

Drug Distribution System

Drugs will be acquired in bulk, stored, mixed, packaged, labeled, and distributed to users on prescription of physicians. This will be done in the drug facility by licensed pharmacists employed by or under contract to the management corporation. Drugs may be furnished to enrollees under a prepayment plan or for cash.

Prescriptions will be filled only on physicians' instructions. However, a system will be established to change proprietary names to their equivalent generic designations. At the appropriate time, a pharmacopoeia data system will be prepared to make drug selections, find suitable substitutes, cross-reference trade names with generic designations, and to cost prescriptions.

Patient Logistics System

Patients will come to the center in their automobiles, on public transportation, or by transportation of the center. It is planned that a car pool will be operated by the center's personnel or volunteers. Also, a mini-bus system is envisioned throughout East Windsor to serve incapacitated patients, or those who don't drive. Parking space will be provided at facilities.

All patients will check in at the reception desk. General inquiries will be handled by the receptionist; potential enrollees will be routed to the administrative office. Emergency cases will be sent to the emergency facility; those requiring tests, therapy, physician consultation, etc., will be routed to the proper centers.

A general waiting room will be available at the reception area with secondary areas in service centers as needed. Adequate facilities for patient comfort, washrooms, reading materials, play area, etc. will be provided. The procedure for handling patients in each service area will be left to practitioners with the advice of the administrative staff to conserve space.

CONTROL SYSTEMS

Special care will also be given to creation of the following control systems:

1. Policy control system.
2. Overall performance evaluation system.
3. Family health management system.
4. Quality control system.
5. Accounting system.
6. Data processing system.

Policy Control System

Policy of the center will be made by the board of trustees in HMO. The administrator will see that it is carried out and he will report to the board on compliance. Policy will be set at board meetings in accordance with statutory provisions, articles of organization, and bylaws of HMO.

To make sure policy is sound, the board will have trustees representing users, the medical group, and the management group. These trustees will keep informed on problems of those they represent, and procedure will help them do so. For example, a medical committee will consider problems of providers. By committee meetings, each one will have an opportunity to influence policy. Trustees representing the medical committee will bring committee resolutions and observations before the board. In turn, they will explain board action to providers through the committee. A similar mechanism will be set up for the management group.

A special mechanism will get views of users into policymaking. The management corporation will develop, install, operate a consumer opinion system. Users will be polled by query cards in waiting rooms.

Complaints will be funneled into a processing area, analyzed, abstracted, and brought to proper attention. Special surveys will be made of enrollees as occasions arise. Information gathered will be summarized for trustees with details available on request.

Finally, trustees will be given reports and statements on operations and status of the center, including performance evaluation, quality reviews, utilization, and financial reports. They will be apprised of important events, including actual and anticipated changes in primary relationships among major components of the system. The administrator will be responsible for getting this information to trustees in an efficient and timely manner.

Overall Performance Evaluation System

A system will be devised to measure overall performance of the center. It will compare goals with accomplishment. Goals will involve health status of the community, services rendered, quality of service, cost, utilization of facilities, and consumer satisfaction.

Goals and budgets will be set annually by the trustees with support of the management group. They will be made known to all concerned as events occur; statistics bearing on goals will be compiled, such as illness incidents, procedures administered, hospital bed days, etc. Public health statistics also bearing on goals will be accumulated, and when needed, surveys will be made to measure the health progress in the community. These figures, with others on quality and consumer satisfaction, will be processed to provide performance values commensurate with goals. The information will be summarized and reported to trustees periodically.

Family Health Management System

The management group will establish and operate a system to help enrollees manage their own health maintenance. Initiative for seeking curative care will be largely up to the user. Guided by education, users will phone for appointments when feeling ill or experiencing symptoms. Once the patient enters the system, it will be up to the center to guide him and see that he receives proper care until his discha rge. The care will largely be controlled by traditional physician-patient procedures. However, when a patient's regular doctor is unavailable or he has no regular doctor, the administrative group will make the proper care relationships.

Initiative for other care will start with the center. Enrollees will be notified by bulletin or letter about inoculations, special screenings, educational classes, etc. Preventive treatment, such as periodic physicals, will be prescribed by physicians for every enrollee, and the administrative department will schedule and follow up on routines prescribed. Critical therapy and treatment will be scheduled in like manner.

Logs will be kept of all entries into the system and of treatment rendered. Critical schedules will be entered into patients' files, compliance recorded, and noncompliance listed for follow up. As necessary, follow up will be done by mail, telephone and home visits depending on the circumstances.

Quality Control System

A system for controlling quality of medical care will be designed, installed, and operated by the medical group with assistance of the administrative department. Quality will be controlled by peer review. Standards for working conditions, provider qualifications, volumes of services to be rendered, types of services, procedures, measurement standards, degrees of accuracy, and standards for the maintenance of medical records will be established. Surveys will be made to compare actual practice with standards. Periodically an audit will be made of each practice to check conformance with quality standards; reports will be prepared and entered into the center's files. Deviations from standards will be presented to each practitioner responsible, and continued deviations will be cause for terminating relationships with the center.

A suitable outside agency will be employed to make periodic independent audits of the quality control system. It will review procedures, analyze case histories, and render opinions on adequacy of quality control.

In the event of a dispute concerning quality, impartial arbiters will be appointed to consider the matter and render a decision which will be binding on all parties.

Accounting System

The accounting system will be a group of independent but interrelated systems. Each organization of the center will have its own records and reports which will be consolidated for an aggregate picture of total operations. Accounting for HMO and the management corporation will be done by the administrative department. Participating practitioners can choose to do their own accounting or have it done for them by the administrative department.

HMO accounting will consist largely of posting and summarizing capitation receipts, provider charges, and payments. Each service charge will be compiled by both enrollee and provider accounts. Source documents will contain procedure codes, patient descriptors, provider codes, and other data required for cost and price analysis. Ledger accounts will be kept and reports prepared to give a well rounded assortment of financial summaries and operating statements.

Accounting of the management corporation will consist of posting and summarizing source records of charges, cash sales, receipts, payroll, purchases, accrued charges, and payments. Source documents will be coded by a chart of accounts to provide statistical analysis of income expenditure, unit costs, and performance data. Financial statements will be prepared monthly, including departmental performance reports.

Practitioners will be responsible for their own accounting methods and their records should be good enough to show clearly revenues and expenditures for services rendered. In addition, practitioners will be encouraged to adopt uniform accounting and use accounting services of the management corporation.

Data Processing System

A linked data system will be devised and adopted progressively. It will consist of a standardized line item module, coding systems, and compatible records. The module will be capable of generating information items for all transactions and status situations, items easy to manipulate that are machine readable, and compatible with one another. For example, a service transaction in a provider center should generate a line item that can be used for billing, overhead distribution, statistical analysis, etc.

Coding systems will be devised for service centers, procedures, types of transactions, users, etc.

Records will accomodate the standardized modules of information. They will be compatible with one another in format, timing, and media used and standardized sufficiently to be compatible with common information processing equipment such as typewriters, bookkeeping machines, and electronic data processing equipment.

Electronic data processing will be used where it is economical. In-house, service bureau, and time sharing equipment will be considered for booking, billing, bookkeeping, patient records, diagnostic analysis, drug reference, procedure look-up, and others.

Facilities Plan

Facilities will be acquired to accommodate the planned systems of operation. Land, buildings, and equipment will be purchased or rented as required. Since most of the facilities needed are already available, the plan is to build around them.

Several sites are available in East Windsor. The primary facility is the professional building owned by Hightstown Associates. Located on One Mile Road Extension in the western half of the township, it has 8,500 square feet on a three acre tract. Some 2,500 feet are not yet completed, but will be completed to serve as part of the center. The building is ideally located in the growth area of the western half of the township it has 8,500 square feet on a three-acre tract. Some 2,500 feet are not yet completed, but will be completed to serve as part of the center. The building is ideally located in the growth area of the western half of the township and less than one mile from a planned township center to be constructed in later years.

Other possible sites are professional centers elsewhere in the township. One site will have two adjoining buildings totalling 16,000 square feet. One of the buildings is nearing completion, the other will be started in the near future. The site is in the heart of the shopping area of Twin Rivers, with plenty of parking available.

These sites could be acquired for the center. They are available for rent or purchase. The space contained, 24,500 square feet, is enough for the foreseeable future; and there is room for expansion. Parking space is ample. The buildings can be modified to meet specifications with a minimum of investment.

The facilities will house HMO, the management corporation, and the medical group. They will contain reception areas, professional suites for physicians, dentists, therapists, X-ray facilities, an educational center, diagnostic center, an emergency area, laboratory space, drug dispensary, administrative space, and general service areas. Layout will be flexible and expandable. Facilities will handle service volumes, striking an economic balance between service levels and costs to provide them.

Equipment required, estimated at $300,000 initially, will be determined and acquired. Physicians and dentists are expected to provide their own furniture and movable professional equipment. Major X-ray and other equipment will be furnished by a contract provider. Other equipment will be furnished by the center, for the emergency facility, diagnostic center, education department, administrative department, and general services. The following rough estimate has been made of new equipment requirements by usage center:

Education	$ 10,000
Administration	30,000
Transportation	15,000
Diagnostic Center	20,000
Emergency Center	25,000
Total	$100,000

Decisions to rent or purchase will be made as requirements are finalized and financing alternatives are examined. For planning purposes, it is assumed that all but about $100,000 of equipment will be rented and that one-half of the amount to be purchased will be financed by grants.

Fiscal Plan

The medical center will become financially self-sufficient at an early time. Funds for operation will come from payers for medical services. During early operation, most funds will be paid directly from patients to providers on a fee-for-service basis. As people become enrolled in the plan, revenues will flow from payers to HMO through the fiscal intermediary (HFI).

The system will therefore provide for a primary flow of funds through the fiscal intermediary with a supplemental flow from patient to physician for the near future. The intermediary will deduct administrative costs and cost of catastrophic insurance from funds received, and the remainder will be paid to HMO on a capitation basis. A reserve will be maintained by the intermediary to smooth chance variations in receipts and expenses.

After receiving capitation payments, HMO will redistribute funds to providers of care, HMC, employees, and suppliers out of a pool which will also include rents collected for buildings and equipment. It will keep a reserve to smooth fiscal fluctuations and will share surpluses and deficits with the fiscal intermediary and providers in the prepayment plan.

The individual members, partners, and corporations that make up the medical group, HMG, will receive revenues from HMO on a fee-for-service formula basis and will collect fees directly from non-enrolled patients. They will use these funds to reimburse themselves, staff, and suppliers, and HMO for facilities rented.

The management corporation (HMC) will receive fees from HMO for services and from patients who elect to pay for their own prescriptions and laboratory tests. These sums will be distributed to employees, suppliers and stockholders of HMC.

Exhibit 16 is a matrix which illustrates anticipated flow of funds in the system at a time when it has 20,000 enrollees with full prepayment coverage. The illustration assumes constant dollars and realistic assumptions on how revenue will divide among different providers.

Reading down the chart, payers would put out $5.4 million annually with $5.2 million going to HMO via the intermediary and $0.2 million directly to HMC for cash sales. The intermediary in turn would remit $5.0 million to HMO, keeping $0.2 million for its own account.

HMO, receiving $5.0 million from the intermediary and $160 thousand from the medical group for rent would pay out $1.7 million to the

---

EXHIBIT 16
Fiscal Projections
$ 000 Annually

TO	Payers	HFI	FROM HMO	HMG	HMC	TO TOTALS
HFI	$5,200					$ 5,200
HMO		5,000		160		5,160
HMG			1,700			1,700
HMC	200		750			950
Intermediary Resources		200				200
House Professionals				1,100		1,100
Contract Providers			2,525			2,525
HMX Employees			20	340	300	660
HMX Suppliers & Others			165	100	460	725
Internal Revenue Service					90	90
Private Investors					100	100
FROM TOTALS	$5,400	5,200	5,160	1,700	950	$18,410

Note: Based on 100% prepayment involving 20,000 enrollees in
         1972 $s.

medical group, $750 thousand to the management corporation, $2.525 million to outside providers, $20 thousand to employees, and $165 thousand to suppliers.

The medical group, out of $1.7 million received, would pay $160 thousand to HMO for rent, $1.1 million to professional staff, $340 thousand to employees, and $100 thousand to suppliers.

Out of the $950,000 received by the management group, $300,000 would go to employees; $460,000 to suppliers; $90,000 to taxes; and $100,000 to investors.

Overall Program

The Hightstown project will be continued until the proposed system is operational. Advanced planning will be conducted in the first two quarters; implementation in the subsequent three quarters. Operations will be self-sufficient in about 15 months. Exhibit 17 is a tentative schedule for the overall program.

During the first quarter, additional sponsors will be sought to support the project, legal research will be completed, and working arrangements set up with cognizant government agencies. Also in this quarter, providers will be lined up, the benefits package finalized, a fiscal intermediary chosen, enrollees recruited, and systems designed.

In the second quarter, a health audit will be made of all prospective enrollees, facilities will be designed, the financial plan established, the organization completed, financial arrangements completed, and building contracts made.

In the third quarter, construction will be done, HMC organized, key people recruited, facilities occupied, and installation of systems begun.

In the fourth quarter, systems installations will be completed, and operations started.

In the fifth quarter, the operation will be shaken down.

Zero date for commencing this schedule will be the date advanced planning funds are received from the Department of Health, Education, and Welfare.

Resources needed are listed in Exhibit 18. They are catalogued by component organization: HMO, the medical group, and the management corporation.

For HMO, one-half time of the president is needed for two quarters, and one-fourth time thereafter. A full-time administrator and three assistants are required for the first six months and part-time of the administrator and one assistant thereafter. Full-time services of several

EXHIBIT 17
Overall Project Schedule

LEGEND		1st Qtr	2nd Qtr	3rd Qtr	4th Qtr	5th Qtr
				QUARTER		
HMO	Hightstown Medical Organization	1	1	1	1	1
LWYRS	Legal Counsel	2		16		
CONSLTS	Consultants	3		17		
ADM	Administrator of HMO	4	4	18		
STAFF	Staff of HMO	5	5	19		
LAB	Contract Laboratory	6	6	20	20	
ENG	Engineering Contractor	7	7		21	
		8	8		22	22
		9	9			
			10			
			11			
			12			
			13			
			14			
			15			

No.	Tasks	Performer	No.	Tasks	Performer
1	Get sponsors	HMO	12	Refine financial plan	ADM & CONSLTS
2	Do legal research	LWYRS	13	Realign organization	ADM & CONSLTS
3	Make agency arrangements	CONSLTS	14	Close financial contracts	ADM & CONSLTS
4	Line up providers	ADM & CONSLTS	15	Close building contracts	ADM & CONSLTS
5	Create benefits package	ADM & CONSLTS	16	Supervise construction	ADM & CONSLTS
6	Get fiscal intermediary	ADM & CONSLTS	17	Organize HMC	ADM & CONSLTS
7	Negotiate benefits contracts	ADM & CONSLTS	18	Recruit key people	ADM & CONSLTS
8	Line up enrollees	STAFF	19	Move into facilities	ADM & CONSLTS
9	Design systems	STAFF & CONSLTS	20	Install systems	ADM & CONSLTS
10	Make health audit	LAB	21	Start operations	ADM & CONSLTS
11	Design facilities	ENG	22	Shake down operations	ADM & CONSLTS

consultants are needed for the first six months. In addition, 10,000 feet of floor space and room for 80 cars will be needed in the third quarter, increasing to 20,000 feet and room for 200 cars in the fifth year. Finally, to acquire these resources, funds will be needed: $170,000 for advanced planning in the first two quarters, and $100,000 to purchase equipment in the third quarter.

For the medical group, fifteen providers are needed at the beginning with the support of 30 other employees. By the fifth year, HMG's requirements will expand to 25 providers and 50 others.

For the management group, approximately 10 employees will be required in the third quarter with additions continuously until the fifth year when 20 to 25 people will be needed. To support these people at the beginning, start-up capital amounting to $150,000 will be needed in the third quarter.

EXHIBIT 18
Resource Requirements

Items	Measure	1st Qtr	2nd Qtr	2nd Half	2nd Yr.	5th Yr.
HMO						
President	Number	1/2	1/2	1/4	1/4	1/4
Administrator*	Number	1	1	1/4	1/4	1/4
Adm. Assts.*	Number	3	3	1/4	1/4	1/4
Land	Acres			2	2	2
Parking Space	Cars			80	120	200
Building Space	Sq. Ft.			10,000	15,000	20,000
Plng. & Facility Funds	($000)	85	85	100		
Consultants	Number	3	2			
Enrollees	Number			2,000	6,000	20,000
Medical Group						
Physicians and Dentists	Number			15	20	25
Nurses and Others	Number			30	40	50
Management Corp.						
Administrator*	Number			3/4	3/4	3/4
Adm. Assts.*	Number			3-3/4	4-3/4	5-3/4
Residents	Number			1	1	2
Parameds	Number			1	2	2
Pharmacists	Number			1	3	4
Lab Techs.	Number			1	3	4
Custodian	Number			1	1	1
Drivers	Number			1	1	2
Educators	Number			1	1	2
Consultants	Number			2	1/2	—
Operating Funds	$			150		

*Administrator and one assistant will work for both HMO and Management Corp. After Management Corp. is created, other 2 administrative assistants will be transferred there.

Financial Plan

The plan calls for $1,460,000 of capital to get the system started and financially independent. A breakdown of capital requirements is as follows:

Seed money	$ 40,000
Development funds	170,000
Land & buildings	800,000
Equipment	300,000
Venture capital	150,000
Total	$1,460,000

An initial expense of about $30,000 has been incurred for concept and early planning phases of the project. This initial expense was incurred by Hightstown Medical Organization and indirectly by others who have waived or deferred payment for services. It is planned to reimburse those who deferred payment out of sponsorship funds amounting to $40,000 which will be raised later.

Plans call for raising sponsorship funds as the prepayment plan gets under way. Sponsorship bonds paying an annual rate of interest will be offered to plan providers as they join the center, redeemable when they leave it. Funds amounting to $170,000 will be acquired from HEW by application under Public Law 89-749. These funds will be used for development.

Land and buildings valued at approximately $800,000 are available for lease or purchase. Approximately $500,000 has been invested in these facilities, $300,000 by Hightstown Medical Associates and $200,000 by Twin Rivers; and around $300,000 more has been budgeted for completing the facilities.

Equipment estimated at $200,000 will be furnished by physicians and other providers for their own individual use. Another $100,000 will be provided by the center for its emergency facility, diagnostic area, administrative offices, and so forth. Some $100,000, needed to procure equipment, will be raised by grant application under Hill-Burton and by an FHA guaranteed loan secured by sponsorship funds. In this phase of the financing, goals may be raised to get additional funds for possible escalation of requirements.

An amount of $150,000 will be needed to start up operations. Since the medical group will consist of providers who begin with large practices, no start-up capital will be required for it; and since HMO will have a small staff getting administrative support from the management corporation, no start-up capital will be required for it, except for the seed money previously mentioned. The management corporation, however, will need $150,000 for staff expenses until it can reach a break even point.

Venture capital for start-up will be raised by corporate financing instruments from either private individuals, a banking house, a small business investment corporation, or other source. If pending legislation goes through in time, a 90% loan guarantee will be sought. Otherwise, a proposition will be prepared with terms sufficiently attractive to get needed capital. Propositions, already drawn up and explored, will be refined and presented in prospectus form to potential investors. Tax shelters and other attractive features will be exploited to raise funds.

The plan for raising venture capital is designed with several safety factors. It calls for twice the capital that would be required if everything should go well. Further, the profitmaking potential of the management corporation, while not large, is enough to attract several times the start-up capital needed. Finally, a fund raising drive will be made if private financing is insufficient.

Exhibit 19 summarizes financial projections for HMO and the management corporation. The first two parts are for HMO, the second two for HMC. Part 1 projects the revenue and expenses of HMO. It shows development grant income for the past two quarters and how it will be spent, and shows operating income with expenses thereafter. Part 2 shows balances and cash flow for HMO. Part 3 presents projected income and expenses of the management corporation: revenues from HMO and others, how the proportion of payments changes as the prepayment plan gets under way, and expenses of employees providing educational services, diagnostic tests, drugs, and administrative support. It also shows operating profit and loss indicating when the operation will break even and how much it will earn as it gets under way. Part 4 summarizes operating profits for the management corporation, makes tax estimates, projects net profits and shows balances and cash flow projections.

ADVANCED PLANNING DETAILS

The advanced planning part of the overall program will be conducted in six months following acceptance of the grant application to HEW. The goal of the program is to prepare the components of the proposed medical system for start-up operations. The program should not only pave the way to a successful operation, but should demonstrate that an HMO can be created in a short time with minimal

EXHIBIT 19-1
Financial Projections—Hightstown Medical Organization
($000)

Items	1st Qtr	2nd Qtr	2nd Half	2nd Yr.	3rd Yr.
Grant Income	$72	98			
Operating Revenues			250	1,000	2,000
Rental Income			40	120	160
Total Income	72	98	290	1,120	2,160
Payroll	15	20	10	20	20
Office Space Rental	1	1	2	4	4
Services & Supplies	2	2	2	4	4
Depreciation			5	10	10
HMG-Payments			80	330	660
HMC-Payments			40	150	300
Contract Provider Payments			125	490	1,000
Facility Rental			35	105	140
Interest Payments			3	7	7
Consulting	25	30			
Legal	10	10			
Engineering		10			
Promotion Materials	5	10			
Other Development Expense	14	15			
	72	98	302	1,120	2,145
Surplus/Deficit	—	—	(12)	—	15

EXHIBIT 19-2
Financial Projections—Hightstown Medical Organization
($000)

Items	1st Qtr	2nd Qtr	2nd Half	2nd Yr.	3rd Yr.
BALANCES					
Cash	$		2	9	31
Facilities	=	=	95	85	75
Total	=	=	97	94	106
Loans	—	—	64	81	78
Payables	20	20	20	—	—
Surplus/Deficit	(20)	(20)	13	13	28
Total	=	=	97	94	106
CASH FLOW					
Facilities Grant			45		
Bank Loan*			45		
Loans**			20	20	
Operating Receipts	72	98	340	1,120	2,160
Total Received	72	98	450	1,140	2,160
Facilities Expenditure			100		
Bank Loan Repayment			1	3	3
Operating Disbursement	72	98	347	1,130	2,135
Total Disbursed	$72	98	448	1,133	2,138

* 10 years @ 9%.
**Indefinite @ 10%.

EXHIBIT 19-3
Financial Projections—Management Corp.
($000)

Items	3rd Qtr.	4th Qtr.	2nd Yr.	3rd Yr.	4th Yr.	5th Yr.
Received from HMO	$ 15	25	150	300	500	750
Received from Patients	35	75	450	400	300	200
Total Income*	50	100	600	700	800	950
Administrator (3/4)	4	4	16	16	16	16
Adm. Assts.	10	10	40	48	48	48
Residents	4	4	16	16	32	32
Parameds	4	4	16	32	32	32
Pharmacists	4	8	40	40	55	55
Lab Techs.	3	5	30	30	30	30
Custodian	3	3	12	12	12	12
Drivers			6	12	12	12
Educators	4	4	16	16	16	30
Consultants	24	24	24	22	25	27
Fringe Benefits	4	5	20			
Drugs	8	15	90	105	120	140
Outside Lab Tests & X Ray	10	20	120	140	160	190
Office Rentals	4	4	16	18	20	20
Equipment Rentals	4	4	16	18	20	20
Supplies & Other	5	10	60	70	80	95
Interest	3	3	11	9	7	4
Total Expense	98	127	539	604	685	763
Operating Profit/Loss	$(48)	(27)	61	96	115	187

*Income make up: Screening-40%, Tests-10%, Drugs-30%, Education & Protection-10%, Other Services-10%.

EXHIBIT 19-4
Financial Projections—Management Corp.
($000)

Items	3rd Qtr.	4th Qtr.	2nd Yr.	3rd Yr.	4th Yr.	5th Yr.
Gross Income	$(48)	(27)	61	96	115	187
Income Taxes	—	—	—	35	51	87
Net Income	(48)	(27)	61	61	64	100
BALANCES						
Cash	104	73	106	118	101	109
Accounts Receivable	10	15	25	50	75	100
Total	114	88	131	168	176	209
Accounts Payable	10	16	24	28	32	38
Loans*	144	137	111	83	53	20
Equity	(40)	(65)	(4)	57	91	151
Total	114	88	131	168	176	209
CASH FLOW						
Paid In Capital	10					
Loans	150					
Operating Receipts	40	95	590	675	775	925
Total	200	95	590	675	775	925
Dividends					30	40
Loans Repaid	6	7	26	28	30	33
Operating Disbursements	90	119	531	635	732	844
Total	96	126	557	663	792	917

*5 Years @ 8%.

subsidies. Further, it should demonstrate that an HMO can have features prescribed by HEW and still be attractive to both physicians and patients. Finally, it should demonstrate that start-up costs and the consequent hazard of failure can be kept to a minimum by an evolutionary approach to prepayment which allows a mixing of capitation with prepayment as the plan evolves.

Advance planning tasks will be performed in five general areas of endeavor:

A   Establishment of Key Relationships.
B   Development of the Benefits Package.
C   Preenrollment.
D   Design of Organization, Systems, & Facilities.
E   Financing of Construction & Start- Up.

Exhibit 20 is a list of advanced planning tasks to be performed; Exhibit 21 a schedule for performing them; and Exhibit 22 a summary of projected advanced planning costs.

Key Relationships

The first set of tasks is to establish relationships with outside agencies, providers, and employees. Scheduled for the first sixteen weeks, tasks are:

1. Legal Research.
2. Establish Working Relationships with the Public.
3. Line-Up of Providers.
4. Employment of Key Staff.

Legal Research

This task includes a study of statutory, professional, commercial, and financial limitations to the planned system, a description of obstacles that might be encountered, recommendations on handling difficulties, and legal opinions on critical issues not easily resolved. Some of the problems to be explored are whether the center qualifies as an HMO under state law, whether it can get a certificate-of-need, and whether it can join together in one center the variety of medical

---

EXHIBIT 20
Advanced Planning Tasks

A.   Establish External Relationships:

  1. Perform legal research to determine statutory and other limitations.

  2. Establish working relationships with cognizant local, state, and federal agencies.

  3. Line up physicians, dentists, and other providers of medical care.

  4. Recruit key staff members for the project team.

B.   Develop the Benefits Package:

  1. Finalize the medical services to be provided initially.

  2. Complete actuarial studies to establish rates.

  3. Contract with the fiscal intermediary.

C.   Enroll Recipients of Care:

  1. Negotiate benefits contracts with "payors": federal and state agencies, industries, and unions.

  2. Recruit enrollees.

  3. Conduct health audit of enrollees.

D.   Design Organization, Operating Systems, and Facilities:

  1. Realign organization as necessary to meet HEW requirements.

  2. Design internal operating systems.

  3. Design control systems.

  4. Design necessary facilities. Prepare equipment requirements and facilities layouts.

E.   Secure Construction and Start-up Financing:

  1. Refine preliminary financial plans as required.

  2. Locate investors: private investors and possible government sources of funds.

EXHIBIT 21
Advanced Planning Schedule

Tasks	Responsibility	Man-months	Elapsed Weeks Start Week	Elapsed Weeks Complete Week
A. Relationships				
1. Legal research	Legal Counsel	1.0	0	12
2. Agency relationships	Consultants	1.0	0	8
3. Line up providers	Adm/Cnslts	2.0	0	16
4. Recruit key staff	Adm/Cnslts	1.0	0	8
B. Benefits Package				
1. Finalize benefits package	Adm/Cnslts	1.0	0	16
2. Payment plan	Adm/Cnslts	2.0	9	26
3. Get intermediary	Adm/Cnslts	1.0	0	16
C. Pre-Enrollment				
1. Negotiate benefits package	Adm/Cnslts	1.0	9	26
2. Recruit enrollees	Adm/Staff	4.0	9	26
3. Make health audits	Staff/Cont Lab	1.0	9	26
D. Organization, Systems, and Facilities				
1. Realign organization	Leg. Cnsl/Cnslts	2.0	16	26
2. Design support systems	Staff/Cnslts	2.0	0	26
3. Design control systems	Staff/Cnslts	3.0	0	26
4. Design facilities	Adm/Engr	1.0	13	26
E. Financing				
1. Refine financing plan	Adm/Cnslts	1.0	16	26
2. Find financial support	Adm/Cnslts	2.0	16	26
A. to E. Monitoring of Project and Preparation of Final Report	Adm/Staff	4.0	26	36

EXHIBIT 22
Advanced Planning Cost Projections

Tasks		Estimated Costs
A.	Relationships	
	1. Legal research	$ 5,000
	2. Agency relationships	5,000
	3. Line up providers	15,000
	4. Recruit key staff	5,000
B.	Benefits Package	
	1. Finalize benefits package	5,000
	2. Payment plan	10,000
	3. Get intermediary	5,000
C.	Pre-Enrollment	
	1. Negotiate benefits package	5,000
	2. Recruit enrollees	25,000
	3. Make health audits	25,000
D.	Organization, Systems, and Facilities	
	1. Realign organization	15,000
	2. Design support systems	10,000
	3. Design control systems	15,000
	4. Design facilities	10,000
E.	Financing	
	1. Refine financing plan	5,000
	2. Find financial support	10,000
	Total Costs	$ 170,000

Advanced Planning Costs by Resource

Project Staff	12 man-months	$ 20,000
Staff Overhead		20,000
Consultants	15 man-months	55,000
Legal Counsel	2 man-months	20,000
Civil Engineers	1 man-month	5,000
Laboratory Services		25,000
Promotional Materials		15,000
Travel and Related Expenses		10,000
Total Costs		$ 170,000

services proposed. Other questions pertain to the prepayment plan and how it conforms with insurance regulations, to liability of providers under the plan and how exposure can be minimized, and to potential fair practice disputes under commercial law and professional regulations. This work will be performed and completed by attorneys in approximately 12 weeks at a cost of around $5,000.

Working Relationships with the Public

This task will create relationships with the local community, state agencies, federal agencies, trade associations, unions, professional societies, and others of a public or quasi-public nature who may influence the system. The parties will be identified, approached, briefed, and engaged. Working relationships will be created with groups such as local planning councils, committees on health improvement, public health agencies, A and B health planning agencies, the state Hill-Burton agency, and cognizant departments of HEW. Work will be performed by the acting project manager during the first eight weeks with staff assistance at a cost of approximately $5,000.

Line-up of Providers

This task will get providers interested in working with the medical center. Brochures and other documentation will be prepared to demonstrate the advantages. Physicians, dentists, and others will be sought to join the capitation plan. Hospitals, extended care facilities, specialists in medical care will all be approached to work out service relationships. The administrator of HMO will spearhead this work with the assistance of consultants, and it is expected that most of the potential providers will be lined up within sixteen weeks at a cost of around $15,000. Much printed documentation will be needed to demonstrate programs to potential plan members, including how they will interface with the center, what they will be responsible for, the support they will get, how they will be reimbursed, etc.

Employment of Key Staff

This task will be to recruit an administrator for the center, an executive assistant, and other personnel for the program. Job descriptions and personnel specifications will be prepared, interviewees sought, references checked, and employment agreements reached with successful candidates who will be indoctrinated, and assigned duties. Work will be done by the consultants with assistance of the administrator. It will take up to twelve weeks at a cost of approximately $5,000.

Benefits Package Development

The second set of tasks will develop the benefits package into a prepayment plan ready for implementation by a fiscal intermediary. Work will include the following tasks performed over the full development period of 26 weeks:

1. Benefits Package Completion.
2. Payment Plan Finalization.
3. Intermediary Selection.

Benefits Package Completion

This task will develop the benefits package to the point of costing and pricing. Present coverages will be explored, consumer preferences determined, alternative options conceived and tested, local experience factors accumulated. This package will be refined, defined, and described. It will be presented to interested parties for endorsement and approval. This work will be performed by the administrator and consultants in the first sixteen weeks at a cost of $5,000.

Payment Plan Finalization

This task will develop the payment plan into contractual documents for providers, users, and a fiscal intermediary. Alternative plans will be explored and acceptance tested. Usage and cost factors will be compiled, actuarial analysis made, and contract terms defined through close collaboration with one or more potential intermediaries. Results of a health audit described below will furnish vital inputs for this work. Finally, contractual forms will be drafted. This work will be performed by the administrator, consultants, and legal counsel from the 9th to the 26th week at a cost of $10,000.

Intermediary Selection

This task will result in a contract with a fiscal intermediary. Work already started will be completed. Potential intermediaries will be identified and approached. The plan will be explained and reactions to it sought. Bids will be solicited and evaluated. References will be checked, negotiations conducted, and agreements made. This work will be performed during the first sixteen weeks by the administrator with consulting support at a cost of approximately $5,000.

Pre-Enrollment Tasks

The third group of tasks will set the stage for later enrollment of individuals. Scheduled for the 9th to 26th week, tasks will include:

1. Benefits Package Negotiations.
2. Line-Up of Potential Enrollees.
3. Health Audit of Potential Enrollees.

Benefits Package Negotiations

This will include identification of potential payer groups, their solicitation, negotiations, and the closing of contracts for services. Approaches will be made to the state Medicaid agency, Social Security Administration, unions, and local industry such as McGraw-Hill, RCA, Kentile, Mettler Instruments, NL Industries, and others. Work will be done by the administrator with consulting support starting in the 9th and ending by the 26th week at a cost of approximately $5,000.

Line-Up of Potential Enrollees

This task includes contacting potential enrollees individually and in groups by phone, mail, house call and in other ways to pre-enroll them and have them take a pre-enrollment physical examination. This work will be done by the administrator and his staff from the 9th to 26th week at a cost of approximately $25,000. Around $10,000 of this amount will be for promotional material, travel, and other items.

Health Audit of Potential Enrollees

This task will get information on the health of potential enrollees for refining plans and costing prepayment. It will include screening the pre-enrollees by a special multiphasic procedure to get essential data at the lowest possible cost. Work will be done by an outside laboratory with its staff starting in the 9th and ending in the 26th week at a cost of around $25,000.

Design of Organization, Systems & Facilities

The fourth set of tasks will provide design detail on organization, construction, and installation of systems. Scheduled for the entire development period, tasks are:

1. Organization Realignment.
2. Service Systems Design.
3. Control Systems Design.
4. Facilities Design.

Organization Realignment

This task includes realignment of the board of trustees, bylaw changes, and policy revision to qualify Hightstown Medical Organization as an HMO. It also includes formulation of organization, job descriptions, personnel specifications, compensation plans, and contracts for providers and employees. Work will be done by consultants and lawyers starting in the 16th and ending in the 26th week at a cost of approximately $15,000.

Service Systems Design

This task includes analysis of proposed service systems, preparation of flow charts, equipment lists, tables of manpower, load patterns and ques, layouts, methods, procedures, and other system detail. Systems design will pertain to education, patient screening, physician services, emergency care, drug distribution, patient logistics and others. Work will be conducted by the staff and consultants throughout the entire project at a cost of approximately $10,000.

Control Systems Design

This task includes analysis of proposed control systems, preparation of flow charts, design of forms, equipment lists, staffing patterns, load patterns, layouts, procedures, programming, and other system detail. Systems will be designed for policy formulation, performance evaluation, long range planning, family health management, quality control, accounting, and data processing. Work will be conducted by the project staff and consultants throughout the entire project at a cost of around $15,000.

Facilities Design

This task includes comparison of available facilities with system space requirements, space planning, determination of additional facilities needed, alteration planning, and compilation of bills of material. Work will be done by the administrator with contractor assistance starting in the 13th and finishing in the 26th week at a cost of approximately $10,000.

Financing of Construction & Start-Up

This fifth set of tasks is to refine financial plans and get financing for construction and start-up. Scheduled for the period starting in the 16th and ending in the 26th week, it will include two tasks:

1. Financial Plan Refinement.
2. Getting Financial Support.

Financial Plan Refinement

This task will refine and supplement existing financial plans using the accounting data of providers, results of pre-enrollment efforts, staffing patterns, and bills of material developed. It will result in a complete set of detailed financial plans for HMO and the management corporation and consolidated statements for the provider groups covering income and expenses, balances, and cash flow. Work will be done by the administrator and consultants from the 16th to the 26th week at a cost of approximately $5,000.

Getting Financial Support

This task will involve identification of financial sources, preparation of alternative financial approaches, determination of instruments to be used, approach to sources, negotiations, preparation of applications, and closing of contracts. Work will be done by the administrator with assistance of consultants starting the 16th and ending the 26th week at a cost of approximately $10,000.

Time & Cost

The advanced planning tasks will be completed as scheduled within cost estimates. To assure this, the schedule shown in Exhibit 21 will be elaborated and cost estimates in Exhibit 22 will be exploded as necessary for monitoring purposes. Overall completion time is set at 26 weeks. As indicated, many of the projects will be performed in parallel by the administrator, his staff, management consultants, outside legal counsel, civil engineers, outside lab people, and so forth. The part that each will play will be detailed at the start and refined as the project develops.

Overall cost is estimated at $170,000. This amount detailed above by task involves around 30 man-months of work provided by approximately nine people who will enter and leave the project at various times. A summary of expected costs is as follows:

Project staff including overhead	$ 40,000
Consultants & engineers	60,000
Legal counsel	20,000
Outside services and materials	50,000
Total	$170,000

To insure success, a project manager will be in charge at all times. Among his duties, he will operate a project monitoring system. With PERT and other scheduling techniques, tasks will be charted and budgets compiled. A system of reporting will be installed and progress will be compared with objectives periodically. Reports on progress with corrective action will be given at regular intervals to management and cognizant government agencies.

SUMMARY

The proposed system will give the people of East Windsor better health care. It should materially improve the economics of health, lowering the cost of disease and treatment while enhancing personal productivity and capacity to enjoy life.

An early successful operation is contemplated, one which will require a minimum of subsidy. Unique features will include low start-up costs, an early break-even point, and flexibility. These features will go a long way toward insuring success, making the plan a low risk one.

The plan is one that patients will like. It gives them a choice of care, including prepayment. They may also choose their primary care physician. But most important, they will be given a superior package of services with prevention as well as cure, and covering them adequately for catastrophic illness.

The plan is attractive to providers. It will give them the advantages of solo practice and added advantages such as the opportunity to work more closely with colleagues, to get the benefit of better facilities and support services, to gain more leisure time, and to enjoy compensation advantages made possible by fringe benefits, tax reduction, and improved estate planning. These advantages are attained without the need of becoming employees or of sacrificing income.

The proposed system will accommodate fee-for-service payments within a broader framework of capitation payment. It will allow the physician to maintain much of his independence and coveted status role. In short, the system is predicated on the assumption that better practice will provide economic gains for all without any one group singled out for sacrifice.

Finally, the new system will demonstrate to other well endowed communities which are medically underserved, how a pushcart, cottage-industry nonsystem can be converted in a relatively short time to an efficient system of health care.

Index

A

Administrative information systems, 97-98
American Association of Foundations for Medical Care of Stockton
  foundation inventory, 58
American Hospital Association (AHA)
  health care corporation plan, 30
American Medical Association (AMA)
  clinic list, 58
  HMO attitude, 53, 54
  Medicredit plan, 30
  preventive care attitude, 190-191
  procedural codes, 128

B

Billing, 9, 83, 91, 97, 99, 110-111
Blue Cross
  New Jersey, 61
Blue Cross-Blue Shield, 63
Boards of trustees
  executive functions, 113
  patient representation, 84, 120
Bureau of Health Planning and Resources Development, 35

C

California Relative Value Scale, 128
Capital financing
  opportunities, 176-182, 194-196
  sources, 131-132, 172-175

Capitation financing. *See* Prepayment financing
Certificates-of-need, 31, 32, 35, 38, 59, 82
Clinical laboratory services
  federal controls, 34
  inhouse, 109, 110
  tests, 3
Columbia Medical Plan, 49
Comprehensive care, 83, 85, 86
Comprehensive care movement, 14-19, 184
Comprehensive Health Care Organizations (CHOs)
  active programs, 45-47
  enrollee costs, 45, 46, 61
  evaluation of success, 47-50
  financing, 41-43
  growth, 24, 25
  market, 81-82
  opportunities, 178
  patient entry, 95
  requirements for self-reliance, 87
  resources, 102
  size projections, 36
  structural model, 37-44, 91, 99, 103-104, 185
  type of care, 37, 84, 94, 95
Comprehensive Health Planning and Public Health Services
  Act of 1966 (P.L. 89-749), 31
Computerization, 8-10, 110-112
Connecticut General, 63
Consulting firms
  opportunities, 180-182
  participation strategy, 64
  role, 111-112, 139-140
Consumers. *See* Patients

D

Data processing, 8-10, 97, 98-99, 110-112
Deaths
    causes, 5, 16, 190
    costs, 15, 16
Dental laboratory services, 109, 110
Development process
    data tables, 201-236
    Hamilton Medical Park Project,
    145-159, 160
    Hightstown Project, 237-398
    implementation, 159-162
    planning, 138-142
    scope, 135-137
    stages, 142-144
Diagnostic x-ray services, 109, 110
Disability
    incidence, 17
Drug distribution, 51

E

Emergency medical care, 95-96, 108
Employee owned corporations, 121
Epstein, Milton, 61
Estate building, 75-77
    See also Retirement plans

F

Facilities
    CHO model, 40-42, 75, 86-87
    construction, 159-161
    tax advantages, 75
Federal government
    controls, 34
    funds, 35, 41, 42, 61, 63, 172, 174, 175
    HMOs, 4, 32, 48, 176, 184-185
    legislation, 30
    medical industry role, 10-14, 25
    nonprofit organization status, 120
    participation strategy, 66, 68
    planning systems, 35
Federal Housing Administration (FHA)
    loan guarantees, 35, 42, 172, 174
Federated organizations
    market type, 81
    practitioner compensation, 127-128
    structure, 44, 112-114, 115

Financial companies
    CHO role, 42-43
    participation strategy, 64
Fiscal intermediaries
    CHO role, 42, 61
Fiscal systems, 97, 123-131
Foundations, 113-114
Fringe benefits, 128-131
    See also Estate building; Retirement
    plans

G

Genessee Valley Health Association, 49
Group Health Association of America, 25,
    47-48
Group Health Cooperative of Puget Sound,
    121
Group practice
    advantages, 71-74, 192-194
    defined, 23-24
    development model, 138-145, 159-162
    disadvantages, 53, 72, 74, 77, 191-192
    financial alternatives, 123-133
    growth, 1, 3, 6, 7, 24, 25, 183-184
    market, 80-86
    operating systems, 93-99
    opportunities, 175-182, 194-196
    opposition, 25
    organizational alternatives, 112-123
    planning tables, 201-236
    pressures for, 7-10
    quality of care, 72
    resources, 86-87, 100-102, 164-175
    service alternatives, 105-109
    structure, 87-93, 112-117
    support services, 109-112, 165-169
    See also Comprehensive Health Care
    Organizations; Health Maintenance
    Organizations

H

Hamilton Medical Park Project
    background, 145-148
    financial evaluation, 153-156, 158-159,
    160
    policy objectives, 149-151
    structure, 151-153, 154, 155, 156,
    157-158

Harvard Community Health Plan, 49
Healthcare Association of Puget Sound, 37
Health care corporations, 30
Health care costs
  annual, 15-16, 18, 19, 85, 189, 190-191,
    192
  government payment, 10, 11, 25, 65
  hospital expenditures, 6-7, 13
  increase, 3, 19-20
  payers, 65
  public response, 22-23
  third party payments, 11
  work-time loss, 18
Health care industry
  changes, 1, 3-19
  future trends, 22-23
  growth, 19-22
  influences, 2
  legislation, 31-33
  pressures, 29-31
  public utility concept, 12, 32
Health care market
  composition, 82-84
  demand, 85-86
  geographical limitations, 81-82
  types of care, 83, 85-68
Health care payers
  participation strategy, 65-68
Health care unit, 91
Health education, 95
Health, Education, and Welfare, Department of (DHEW), 31, 35, 36, 41, 48, 84,
  137, 186
Health Insurance Plan of New York (HIP),
  25, 46-47, 51
Health Maintenance Organization (HMO)
  Act of 1973 (P.L. 93-222), 2, 13, 31-32,
    41, 43-44, 84, 136, 137
Health Maintenance Organizations
  (HMOs)
  American Medical Association attitude,
    30-31
  closed panel, 32, 40, 41
  data system, 99
  fiscal structure, 35-36
  guidelines for development, 33-35
  HMO Act, 2, 13, 31-32, 41, 43-44, 84, 136,
    137
  limitations, 103-104
  nonprofit status, 120

open panel, 32, 40, 41
prepayment financing. 14, 36, 49, 126
resources, 87
support, 4, 25, 176-177
types of care, 83-84
Health Planning Act of 1975, 12, 34
Health plan unit, 91
Highstown Project
  advanced planning, 379, 388-393
  background, 237-246
  capital financing, 248, 380-388
  facilities, 376, 396
  fiscal plan, 377-379, 396-397
  initial planning, 246-248
  medical services, 251, 253-256
  objectives, 248-251, 252, 253
  organization, 263-376, 395-396
  prepayment plan, 256-261, 393-395
  problems, 261-262
Hill-Burton Program, 12, 31, 34, 35
Holding companies, 89
Hospitals
  expenditures, 6-7, 13
  output, 21-22
  participation strategy, 59-62
  revenue, 21
  role changes, 6-7, 11-12
  utilization, 45-46
Housing and Urban Development (HUD)
  health care grants, 42
Hunterdon Medical Center, 61

I

Illness
  costs, 15, 18-19, 190, 192
  incidence, 16-17, 187-188
  work-time loss, 18
Insurance companies
  CHO role, 42
  group practice opportunities, 176-178
  HMO financing, 175
  impact on medical industry, 11
  participation strategy, 62-63
  prepayment plans, 125-126
Integrated organization
  practitioner compensation, 126
  structure, 43, 112, 113, 114, 115
Internal Revenue Service
  tax regulations, 33, 75, 76

Interstudy of Minneapolis
  HMO inventory, 58

K

Kaiser, Henry, 45
Kaiser Construction Company, 45
Kaiser Health Organization, 13, 24, 37,
  45-46, 72
Keogh Act, 33, 76
Keogh plans, 121
Krile Institute, 72

L

Life expectancy, 190
Local governments
  controls, 34
  planning systems, 35

M

Maricopa Foundation for Medical Care, 49
Medicaid, 13, 31, 34
Medical industry. *See* Health care industry
Medical information systems, 97
Medical practice
  career decisions, 56-59
  development, 4-10, 14-19
  federal government influence, 10-14, 25
Medical support systems, 96-97
Medicare, 13, 31, 34, 84
Medi-Comp of Cleveland, 110
Medicredit, 30
Menninger Clinic, 72
Mercer Hospital, 61
Multiphasic screening, 109, 110
Multispecialty groups
  advantages and disadvantages, 106-108
  CHOs, 24, 72
  defined, 24
  patient entry, 83

N

National Advisory Council, 34
National health insurance (NHI), 14, 29, 30
National Health Planning and Resources
  Development Act of 1974 (P.L. 93-641),
  32, 35

Neighborhood Health Associations, 25
Nonprofit organizations, 119-120

O

Outpatient care, 3, 85, 95, 108

P

Paraprofessionals
  delegation of duties, 116
Partnership for Health Program, 31
Patient booking, 9, 91, 98, 99, 108, 111
Patient-doctor relationship, 84, 108, 109
Patient logistics system, 96
Patients
  boards of trustees representation, 84,
    120
  CHO advantages, 73-74
  demand for care, 85-86
  entry, 83, 95, 108-109
  market composition, 82-83, 85
  processing, 96, 108-109
  sources, 84
  visits, 3, 5
Payment
  methods, 124-128
  See also Prepayment financing
Peer review, 98
PERT, 139
Physician-patient relationship. *See* Patient-doctor relationship
Physicians
  accessibility, 7
  advantages of group practice, 74-77,
    192-194
  CHO role, 38, 39, 40, 43, 44, 45
  compensation, 127
  disadvantages of group practice, 191-
    192
  efficiency, 20-21
  group practices, 3, 24
  HMO role, 14
  opposition strategy, 53-56
  opposition to group practice, 25
  participation strategy, 56-59
  primary care, 38, 95, 165
  role changes, 2, 4-6, 7, 11
  tax incentives, 33, 75, 76, 193-194
  See also Medical practice; Solo practice

Physicians' Bill of Rights, 54-55
Planning agencies, 12, 32, 34-35
Practitioners
    compensation, 126-128
    peer review, 98
    primary care, 165
    specialist market, 85
    See also Paraprofessionals; Physicians
Prepayment financing, 14, 36, 42, 49, 124-126
Preventive care
    American Medical Association attitude, 190-191
    benefits, 74-187
    CHOs, 37, 45, 46, 95
Primary care practitioners. *See* Physicians; Practitioners
Primary medical care systems, 93, 94-96
Private industry
    participation strategy, 67-68
    See also Insurance companies
Professional Corporations (PCs), 121
Professional Standards Review Organization (PSRO)
    Amendments of 1972 (P.L. 92-603), 13, 31, 32, 36, 54
Profit sharing, 121, 127, 193
Prudential Insurance, 63
Public Health Service, 34

R

Resources
    basic, 169-175
    captive, 165, 168-169
    processed, 165, 166-167
Retirement plans, 121
    See also Estate building; Keogh plans
Richardson, Elliot, 4, 29, 47
Ross-Loos, 37
Roth, Russell B., 190-191

S

SBICs
    HMO financing, 175

Service unit, 91
Single specialty groups, 72
    advantages and disadvantages, 105-106, 107
    defined, 24
    patient entry, 83
Sloane-Kettering, 72
Small Business Administration
    loan guarantees, 175
Solo practice
    disadvantages, 8, 57
    estate building, 76-77
    future trends, 184
    physician preference, 7
    pressures, 25
Specialized information processing systems, 98-99
Specialty care systems, 96
State governments
    controls, 34
    legislation, 32
    planning systems, 35
Supply/payroll ratio, 8-9
Supply services, 1, 8, 165, 167, 169
Support services, 96-97, 165-167, 169
    alternatives, 109-112
    CHOs, 40
    opportunities, 180
    participation strategy, 63-64

T

Tax advantages, 33, 75, 76, 129, 130, 139, 193-194
Tax exempt status, 120, 130
Tax option corporation, 121

U

United Fund, 13

V

Venture capital, 174-175, 179

About the Author

John Field received his engineering degree from Columbia University, attended the Wharton School of Business and obtained a graduate degree in economics from Columbia University. He has been a consultant to both industry and government. As a principal of a leading consulting firm, he worked with a score of Fortune 200 company presidents on top-level problems and with the Secretary of Defense in unifying the armed services after World War II.

During his career, Mr. Field served as head of his own company, as a senior officer in several giant corporations, as a partner of Peat Marwick Livingston, and was an associate of the late Robert Heller. He has published nearly one hundred articles on business and economics, including the first business-like annual report on the American economy, and a number of monographs on national healthcare markets. In 1969, he headed a study team for Governor Nelson Rockefeller that lead to a cutback in the New York State Medicaid Program which had been getting out of hand. In that study Mr. Field was one of the first to point out both the need and feasibility of providing catastrophic medical insurance for all citizens.

As a freelance consultant, Mr. Field has served as president of a company in the medical services field where he and his staff pioneered the use of computers as a tool of physicians. Other companies for which he served as a consultant are General Electric, Westinghouse, General Dynamics, Cities Service, Carborundum, Bowater, Panhandle Eastern, Kaiser Industries, Continental Can, and Singer.

In addition to his career as consultant, Mr. Field is a faculty member of the New School for Social Research, a consulting editor of *Physician's Management*, and a director of the Advance America Foundation. Recently, he has been a writer and a participant in a weekly television series dealing with the national economic scene.